T0215369

"I have personally acted as a medical malpractice defense expert on numerous occasions. I found that this book clarified my understanding of the medical-legal system and introduced me to entirely new perspectives on the conduct of the expert witness. Whether you are just starting out, or if you are already in this field, you will find this book to be a great resource."

James Aragona, M.D.
Orthopedist

"Where was this gem when I started out as a medical expert 25 years ago? Comprehensive, focused and immediately useful, Mr. Krompier skillfully guides you through the do's and don'ts of expert work. For physicians wading into the medico-legal arena, this is a 'must have'. I heartily endorse this book."

Daryl R. Fanney M.D.
Radiologist

"*Power from Within* is an excellent resource, filling a significant void, for an Expert Witness in the world of medical malpractice defense. It is a comprehensive guide to becoming an expert witness in the medical malpractice arena. The information is accurate, realistic and addresses everything an expert will encounter. I highly recommend this book for anyone who serves as an expert or desires to move into this realm."

Paul M. Greenberg, D.P.M., F.A.C.F.A.S.
Podiatrist

"*Power from Within...* is well-written, concise and easy to understand."

Stephen B. Guss, M.D.
Cardiologist

"Attorney Krompier with more than 30 years of experience in medical malpractice has given us great details and insight into the entire process. This book is a must-read for all physicians and should be part of the medical school or residency curriculum. Having a greater understanding of the medical malpractice process will help to reduce potential frivolous lawsuits. For physicians who are considering being medical defense experts, this book is an excellent guide to a successful and potentially rewarding new endeavor."

John J. Huang, M.D., MBA
Ophthalmologist

"This is a brilliantly written treatise which provides valuable insights into the do's and don'ts of being a successful Medical Malpractice Defense Expert. As someone who has been doing this type of work for nearly two decades, the guidance and advice contained in *Power from Within* is invaluable to a physician beginning his or her expert career, as well as to an experienced expert such as myself. The lessons contained in this work are a recipe for success and, most importantly, help to prevent the common pitfalls encountered when dealing with a cunning plaintiff's attorney. I wish that I could have been guided by such a manual early in my career as a defense expert."

Edward Julie, M.D., F.A.C.C.
Cardiologist

"*Power from Within* by Jeffrey Krompier, Esq. is a must-read for any and all legal defense work to be used by expert witnesses.... The author, a highly experienced certified civil trial attorney, meticulously guides the reader through every step from inception to the finish line. Highly recommend this book. It is the source and reference for a successful journey."

Ezra S. Kazam M.D.
Ophthalmologist

"Mr. Krompier presents a compelling case for physician participation in the medical legal process. He then provides a highly readable, comprehensive, step-by-step, guide full of valuable insights from an attorney's perspective. I recommend it to both novice and seasoned experts."

Mark C. Norris, M.D.
Anesthesiologist

"This is an excellent primer that contains sound, comprehensive guidance for any physician who aspires to be a persuasive expert witness in a medical malpractice case. Written by one of the premier defense lawyers in New Jersey, it covers the entire medico-legal landscape and offers practical, time-tested advice that will benefit anybody engaged in this field. It should be required reading, not only for beginners, but also for veterans."

John O'Farrell
Former trial lawyer, Vice President of
Claims and Legal Consultant to
Princeton Insurance Company

"In *Power from Within*, Jeffrey Krompier has written an outstanding, readable volume designed to help healthcare professionals, from beginners who have never done expert work, to seasoned experts. It focuses on medical malpractice defense consultation, but its wisdom applies to both sides of almost any civil litigation. *Power from Within* covers the whole range from the first discussion with an attorney, to writing expert reports, to testifying effectively at deposition and trial. It offers wisdom applicable to all expert work, and should be required foundational reading for all experts, at all levels of experience."

David Strayer, M.D., Ph.D.
Pathologist

"Indispensable for teaching the novice defense expert the basics as well as honing the skills of the seasoned professional... Essential reading for anyone interested in doing expert malpractice work."

Adam Hecht, M.D.
Radiologist

"This text is a 'must read' for any professional currently doing—or just anticipating doing—expert defense work. I have worked as a malpractice expert for over 25 years, and I agree with all of Mr. Krompier's points. Despite considering myself reasonably experienced, I learned many new things that will help me in future cases."

Charles A. Scott, M.D.
Pediatrician

"The information flowed in such a way that the reader was continually captured by the explanations and examples."

Wendell O. Scott, M.D.
Orthopaedic Surgeon

"Mr. Krompier provides a valuable resource to new and experienced nurses and medical legal experts. This book teaches nurse and physician experts organization skills, the attorney's expectation of the experts and understanding the expert's role. He discusses in detail the potential pitfalls that an expert should avoid as well as proper preparation for court proceedings. Mr. Krompier explains the importance of excellent communication between a nurse or medical expert and the attorney that will lead to a successful case. *Power from Within* is an essential tool for healthcare providers to be thorough and successful nurse and/or medical defense experts."

Paola Vietoris, RN, BSN
Registered Nurse

"This book is a 'must read' for anyone who has or anticipates fulfilling the role of an expert witness. It contains objectives and outlines that assure the reader will develop the skillset needed to be a successful medical malpractice defense expert. The writing style is succinct and the effective use of "do's and don'ts" makes the recognition and acceptance of what needs to be adapted, changed, or retained by the reader readily apparent. The book is superb, I enjoyed reading it."

Desmond A. Jordan, M.D.
Anesthesiologist

"In writing *Power from Within*, Mr. Krompier has done a magnificent job outlining the need and benefits of the defense expert and why they are the key to success in prevailing in medical malpractice litigation. Given the fact that meaningful tort reform is unlikely, *Power from Within* is a game changer and a must-read for every healthcare practitioner because someday they may be litigants themselves and seeking the very best defense expert."

Kenneth Mastria
Claims Manager-Princeton Insurance Co.

"A must-read for any physician contemplating service as a defense expert in medical malpractice cases. Mr. Krompier's insight and experience working with medical experts in medical malpractice litigation is apparent, and a welcomed addition in a sparse field of similar reference materials. This is a very important work that exemplifies the current state of the art and proven strategies for success in and out of the courtroom. His writing style is succinct, clear, and well-tailored to present and share his considerable expertise in this important area. Highly recommended."

Marion R. McMillan, M.D.
Anesthesiologist/Endoscopic Spinal Surgeon

"A masterpiece. As a certified civil trial lawyer, I immediately recognized the value in this writing by Mr. Krompier who is a highly skilled advocate. His insight and effective written communication style provide a road map for the expert witness who seeks to provide meaningful opinions in medical malpractice litigation. In addition to critical instruction on essential preparation for trial, the often overlooked jury perspective, and necessary work commitments from an expert witness, Jeff should be applauded for his unwavering dedication to ethics. He wisely advises that the best experts do not accommodate litigants at the expense of compromising their opinions, thus emphasizing the integrity of the judicial process. A must-read."

Keith J. Roberts, Esq.
Member & Co-Chair, Litigation
Brach Eichler, LLC

"*Power from Within* is the definitive reference source for any physician who is either contemplating serving as a medical defense expert witness or is already a veteran of the process. Drawing from his own career as a dedicated, ethical and highly skilled medical malpractice defense attorney, Jeffrey Krompier has authored a unique and valuable book which cogently and comprehensively summarizes his extensive experience and keen insights in the universe of medical malpractice litigation. The knowledge gained from reading this book is certain to enhance the capabilities and performance of any medical defense expert witness."

Sheldon H. Deluty, M.D.
Anesthesiologist

"This superbly written publication is a jewel for novice and seasoned experts in the field of expert witnesses. Jeff's insights into this field are well organized; his well-articulated guidance provides a valuable asset to expert witnesses of all levels. He meticulously describes the significance of trial preparation, which undoubtedly can be a source of great stress for everyone involved. A must-read!"

Frank Rivera
Claims and Risk Manager

"In our litigious society all physicians practice today with the cloud of malpractice that can negatively affect the ability to treat patients, become a financial and time drain, and hurt one's career and reputation. Mr. Krompier provides a comprehensive, concise and understandable analysis of the entire malpractice process providing insightful guidance on how to successfully defend others as an expert witness. *Power from Within* should be required reading for all physicians, allied health professionals, residents, medical students and hospital executives."

Mark Connolly, M.D.
Cardiovascular Surgeon

"Mr. Krompier, a noted malpractice defense attorney in New Jersey, has written a how-to book on being an effective medical malpractice defense expert that no medical expert involved in these cases should be without. The concepts are clearly stated and well organized. The section on preparing for depositions is particularly notable for all areas one can expect to be questioned about, not just on the opinion. Any new or experienced med-mal expert will benefit from having this volume in their professional reference library."

Carla Rodgers, M.D.
Clinical Associate Professor, Psychiatry

"Excellent introduction to the world of expert witness work. Concisely reviews the requirements, responsibilities, benefits and pitfalls of entering this highly stressful but personally satisfying field. I only wish Mr. Krompier had authored this helpful guide 20 years ago....it would have provided sage advice and saved me much angst during the early years of my medico-legal career."

Adam Elfant, M.D.
Gastroenterologist

"I have been a medical malpractice expert for over two decades, working both plaintiff and defendant cases. Jeffrey Krompier's *Power from Within* has distilled these lessons into a must-read, straight-talk, narrative which anyone who plans to engage in expert work should read. It is even a valuable tool for current veteran experts to improve their performance and to make them even more effective. Overall, very enjoyable and informative."

Gary H. Belt, M.D., F.A.A.N.
Neurologist

"*Power from Within* by Jeffrey A. Krompier, is an excellent guide for any expert physician witness whether experienced or considering to engage in the medical malpractice expert field. I have considered myself mildly experienced but wished I had this book as a reference when I embarked on this journey. I found the book particularly fascinating as it made me reflect on every aspect of this discipline from creating a resume to courtroom demeanor during a trial. In addition, the book provides concrete detailed suggestions in regard to fees especially for novice experts, report writing, sitting in for a deposition and many other steps along the way. Highly recommended."

Wissam Abouzgheib, M.D.
Pulmonary and Critical Care Medicine

"Jeffrey A. Krompier, Esquire's *Power from Within* is an excellent clearly written insightful guide to anyone interested in serving as an expert in the medical malpractice legal system. Jeff provides a very practical outline of the very complex process that often takes place over several years. His many years of experience provide the reader with an honest assessment of what commitment is required from beginning to end."

John A. Russo, M.D.
Internist

"As physicians we are relative fish out of water when we enter the medical legal arena as either defendants or expert medical witnesses. Mr. Krompier's over 30 years of experience as a defense lawyer offers us a comprehensive perspective of the modus operandi and decorum of the medical legal world. His book will assist defendants and experts alike to understand the process and enable us to optimize our function and success in these endeavors. This book will be crucial to medical experts starting out and helpful for seasoned experts who can pick up some insightful pointers. I highly recommend this book to all physicians."

Stephen M. Bloomfield, M.D.
Neurosurgeon

"A comprehensive, authoritative and well-written manual for people contemplating or actively performing medico-legal malpractice testimony. It is highly organized and balanced and covers the process from approaching a case to analyzing the aftermath. I thoroughly enjoyed the book and highly recommend it as an invaluable resource for novice and master witnesses alike. It will refine my effectiveness as a credible expert witness."

Charles M Farber, M.D., PhD
Oncologist

Power from Within

Power from Within
A Guide to Success as a Medical Malpractice Defense Expert

Jeffrey A. Krompier, Esq.

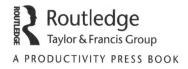

Routledge
Taylor & Francis Group

A PRODUCTIVITY PRESS BOOK

First published 2021
by Routledge
6000 Broken Sound Parkway #300, Boca Raton FL, 33487

and by Routledge
2 Park Square, Milton Park, Abingdon, Oxon, OX14 4RN

Routledge is an imprint of the Taylor & Francis Group, an informa business

© 2021 Taylor & Francis

The right of Jeffrey A. Krompier, Esq. to be identified as author of this work has been asserted by him in accordance with sections 77 and 78 of the Copyright, Designs and Patents Act 1988.

All rights reserved. No part of this book may be reprinted or reproduced or utilised in any form or by any electronic, mechanical, or other means, now known or hereafter invented, including photocopying and recording, or in any information storage or retrieval system, without permission in writing from the publishers.

Trademark notice: Product or corporate names may be trademarks or registered trademarks, and are used only for identification and explanation without intent to infringe.

ISBN: 9780367677374 (pbk)
ISBN: 9780367677381 (hbk)
ISBN: 9781003132608 (ebk)

Typeset in Garamond
by codeMantra

DEDICATION

To my wonderful daughter Alyssa and son Justin.

Contents

Preface

There is no end in sight to the frequency with which physicians, nursing professionals and other healthcare providers will become lawsuit targets in our litigious society. While politicians, practitioners, insurance companies and trial attorneys debate the nation's chronic "malpractice crisis", suits continue to be filed. In addition, once COVID-19 is behind us and the unprecedented public support for health care providers wanes, as it will, it is anticipated that physicians and nurses will become malpractice defendants to a remarkable degree.

National legislative fact-finding committees and investigative bodies, which may be charged with the responsibility of pursuing a solution, likely will never achieve a global remedy. Although curtailed by some states, national legislation has not addressed baseless malpractice suits or grossly excessive monetary verdicts. Another approach exists, however.

Health care providers can impact the existing system and influence the malpractice environment in a tangible, positive and powerful fashion. Although there will be debate over tort reform in order to bring some degree of protection to the malpractice defendant, individual case success, defined from the defendant's perspective as a "no cause" trial verdict, can be realized if well-credentialed and experienced health care professionals are willing to assist the malpractice defense bar as expert witnesses. The benefits to the health care community and the individuals who are willing to participate are innumerable and worth considering.

For more than 35 years, I have represented physicians and nurses in defense of malpractice claims. As a result, I have come to learn that in most instances a lawsuit filed on behalf of an aggrieved patient will rise or fall on the relative success or failure of the liability "expert" retained to testify as to whether the defendant complied with or deviated from the standard of care. Although the surrounding cast of witnesses certainly is important, the cornerstone of a litigant's malpractice case is the liability expert. Ultimately, a jury's decision as to whether a defendant complied with or departed from the standard of care will almost always be based upon expert testimony.

In nearly every malpractice lawsuit, healthcare providers are hired as liability experts for plaintiffs to assist in the identification of facts and issues that will serve as the basis for the advancement of claims against a defendant, the crafting of the Complaint and the matter's ultimate resolution by service as a trial witness. There appears to be no noticeable shortage of practitioners available to plaintiffs in malpractice matters and many are well-credentialed, compelling courtroom witnesses. Although defendants and the defense bar have attracted equally capable practitioners to expert service, more of you should participate.

Over the years, the need for quality malpractice defense experts has persisted. As a result, defense attorneys find themselves repeatedly using the same individuals when circumstances might dictate the need for "new blood". Although retention of the same expert from case to case has some limited advantages, overusing an expert can prove a liability. Defense attorneys would much prefer to have a long list of available and capable experts in every given specialty from which to choose. That is rarely the case.

While universal tort reform would likely be beneficial to the medical and nursing professions, parallel advantages can be realized when quality practitioners devote their energies to service as defense experts. No matter the approach, the purpose is to protect these vulnerable professionals from the "lottery" mentality fueling frivolous lawsuits without arbitrarily twice harming patients with legitimate claims already once injured by "bad care".

Aggressively defended malpractice suits, enhanced by well-credentialed and experienced medical and nursing professionals who are capable of functioning in the legal arena, will increase the likelihood of a defense verdict at trial and send a powerful message to prospective plaintiffs. By offering themselves as defense experts where they should do so—where the merits of the case warrant—practitioners will be part of the solution. Individual lawsuit success enhanced by such service will have a rippling effect. It will give patients and their attorneys pause before unnecessary suits are filed and prompt new thinking by those who might sue when no suit should be contemplated. Thus, serving as a malpractice defense expert cannot only benefit individual colleagues, but such service has the potential long-term and powerful impact of helping to stem the tide of malpractice lawsuits, albeit on a case-by-case basis.

While providing a much needed (and appreciated) service to the profession at large, those of you who participate as malpractice defense experts will be fairly compensated and will enjoy professional rewards. Expert work allows for examination of innumerable practice-related issues. It forces you to stay current on many topics and serves to educate in an exciting way.

Certainly, the mutual gains to be realized both by you and the process in which you participate are important enough to warrant serious thought. Of course, as with any new challenge, the threshold question arises: "Should I do this?" Only you can answer that question. "How do I do this?" This one I'll handle.

Author

Jeffrey A. Krompier, Esq., is the founder and managing partner of the Parsippany, New Jersey, law firm which bears the
name Krompier & Tamn, L.L.C. He is admitted to the bars
of New Jersey and New York. Mr. Krompier is a 1977 magna
cum laude and college honors graduate of Rutgers University
and received both Phi Beta Kappa and Rutgers Scholar des-
ignations. In 1980, Mr. Krompier graduated from Seton Hall
University School of Law, where he was an Associate Articles
Editor of the Law Review and a judicial intern to the late
Honorable Lawrence Whipple of the U.S. District Court for the
District of New Jersey. Upon graduation, Mr. Krompier served
as a judicial law clerk to the late Honorable Bertram Polow of
the New Jersey Superior Court, Appellate Division, and thereafter began the private practice of law. In 1982, Mr. Krompier
joined a medical malpractice defense firm where he practiced
until 1986, when he founded his current firm, which is devoted
to defending healthcare professionals in malpractice matters.

In 1988, the New Jersey Supreme Court certified
Mr. Krompier as a Civil Trial Attorney. Throughout his career,
Mr. Krompier has been recertified five times (1995, 2002,
2007, 2012 and 2017) by the New Jersey Supreme Court as a
Civil Trial Attorney. In 2012, he received certification in Civil
Trial Advocacy by the ABA-accredited National Board of Trial
Advocacy and certification in Civil Pretrial Practice Advocacy

by the ABA-accredited National Board of Civil Pretrial Practice Advocacy. In 2017, Mr. Krompier was recertified in Civil Trial Law and Civil Pretrial Practice Law by the National Board of Trial Advocacy. He is a member of the American Bar Association, American Board of Trial Advocates with Advocate ranking and is a lifetime charter member of Rue Ratings' Best Attorneys of America.

For the last 15 consecutive years (2007–2021), he was named a New Jersey Super Lawyer and has been listed in *Super Lawyers* magazine corporate counsel (2009–2011) and business (2011–2018) editions. In 2014, Mr. Krompier was named an Elite American Lawyer and honored for excellence in the law (2014–2015) by Worldwide Registry. In each of the years 2014 through 2019, he was named one of America's Most Honored Professionals by the American Registry, which also named Mr. Krompier one of America's Most Honored Lawyers in 2020. He also was identified as a Distinguished Attorney by Martindale-Hubbell each year from 2014 through 2021.

In addition, Mr. Krompier is a named expert in the field of medical and dental malpractice defense litigation by Worldwide Who's Who and in 2015 became a lifetime member of Trademark Who's Who Honors Edition. In 2017, he was included in Worldwide Publishing's *Top Lawyers – The Secrets to Their Success*. In 2018, 2019, 2020 and 2021, Mr. Krompier was named one of America's Top 100 High Stakes Litigators for New Jersey and one of America's Top 100 Civil Defense Litigators for New Jersey. In 2021, he was named one of America's Top 100 Medical Malpractice Litigators for New Jersey.

Mr. Krompier is a member of the New Jersey Bar (1980) and the New York Bar (1988) and has been admitted to the U.S. District Court for the District of NJ (1980) and the U.S. Court of Appeals for the Third Circuit (1986). In 2021, Mr. Krompier was admitted to the Bar of the Supreme Court of the United States.

Mr. Krompier has defended in excess of 700 malpractice lawsuits involving most medical specialties and has served as defense counsel in more than 100 malpractice trials from jury selection through verdict.

This is Mr. Krompier's second book. In 2012, he published *Defense From Within – A Guide to Success As a Dental Malpractice Defense Expert* for dental practitioners.

Chapter 1

Introduction— Basic Requirements

Though malpractice defense attorneys and the system in which we function may benefit greatly from your participation, you must understand and accept the demands of defense expert service before deciding to participate.

Time and Flexibility

At a minimum, appreciate that expert service requires time. Even if your interest is genuine, lack of time and the potential for a compromised effort or product will be your undoing and perhaps that of the defendant you intend to help. That said, the amount of time expected or required depends on several factors. Perhaps the most obvious is the amount of work you attract. If you are fortunate enough to receive cases for review at the rate of five to ten per year at the beginning of your "expert" career, and assuming a moderate amount of review material per case (e.g., two to three hospital charts, an equal amount of treaters' office records, two sets of interrogatory answers, four to five deposition transcripts and various miscellaneous documents), it is likely that your otherwise "spare" time will suffice—as in days off, evenings at home or on the weekend. (For an experienced and modestly busy expert receiving 15–20 cases a year, a more significant amount of "spare" time will be needed.)

Equally essential is schedule flexibility. Although reviewing material is central to liability expert service, of equal import are conferences, whether personal, virtual or telephonic. Although you may be able to arrange such confabs around your practice schedule, there will be infrequent occasions when an urgent conference will be dictated by litigation-driven developments. Attorneys who are regularly unable to connect with their experts will become frustrated. Such repeated frustration can only serve to antagonize the attorney, and may have the undesirable and perhaps undeserved effect of altering the otherwise positive perception the attorney has of you. Within the confines of an understandably busy practice, strive to make yourself available.

In addition to document review and conferences, a critical component of liability expert work in many states is the written report. You need to be able to find time not only to scrutinize materials but also to prepare a report in letter form which outlines your review and the opinions derived from that effort. Like document assessment itself, this too is done in your "spare" time ideally and the report can be composed in the comfort of your home, home office or practice office if you prefer. Of course, preparation of the report requires time.

Two exceptions exist to the notion that putting aside time and schedule constraints, you exclusively control all aspects of your effort. Those exceptions are: (1) your deposition (pre-trial testimony), which is not permitted in all jurisdictions; and (2) your trial testimony. Although the deposition may be conducted in your office, your trial testimony rarely is given outside of court, unless required temporarily by COVID-19 limitations. Frankly, if you are unable or unwilling to allow others (judges and attorneys) to play a role in scheduling depositions and trials, you may need to reconsider becoming a malpractice expert.

Depositions can be and often are scheduled at the expert's office. At times, they are conducted at the office of the attorney who has retained you. Site selection is typically the result of agreement between the expert and the retaining lawyer and is based on the expert's convenience, the retaining attorney's convenience, case venue and various other factors. If the matter in which you are participating is located outside your geographic area, you may be asked to travel to a distant deposition site. Alternatively, the deposition in such instances may be conducted by video conference at facilities that offer such services.

COVID-19 has caused depositions to be conducted virtually. It is unclear whether this method will continue once COVID-19 is behind us. However, it is not unreasonable to believe that in some instances, this practice will continue.

Malpractice trials are convened in county (or less frequently federal) courthouses, which will require you to travel. The only exception applies in that instance where your testimony is video-recorded for playback before the jury. As a general rule, most lawyers try to avoid recording an expert's testimony simply because it is not as effective as a live appearance. However, if circumstances dictate this approach, recording typically is done in your office if you have large enough quarters or in the conference room of the retaining attorney. Again, video conference facilities can be used for this purpose, as well as in those instances where you are located in a geographically distant locale.

Once again, COVID-19 restrictions may allow for the use of virtual trial testimony in limited situations. But it remains unclear whether such practice will continue post-COVID-19.

Depositions typically consume two to three hours, exclusive of the pre-deposition meeting with the retaining attorney, which might last one to two hours. Usually, trial testimony in response to both direct and cross-examination will consume

three to four hours. As to both, effective testimony neces-
sitates adequate individual preparation, which itself takes
hours.

Simply and directly stated, you must have and must be
willing to devote time. If you are short on this commodity,
your expert career will be so defined—short.

Communication Skills

The word—spoken and written—is the tool that must be
effectively employed if you are to be successful. Persuasive
communication is critical to the trial attorney who assumes the
responsibility of convincing a jury to support his or her client's
position. An expert must also be able to use language—
technical and lay—effectively.

As mentioned, in many jurisdictions like New Jersey, the
initial product of the liability expert is the "expert report". This
is simply a detailed letter that embodies your opinions. The
contents of the report will be discussed later. For now, understand that the report is prepared after you have reviewed the
materials supplied by the retaining attorney. Once the retaining attorney receives the report, it is supplied to the adverse
attorney where required by the venue's court rules. Since the
expert opinion in a malpractice action is the lynchpin of the
case in almost every instance, the report must address all the
issues essential to the defense and it must be concisely and
convincingly drafted.

Similarly, effective verbal communication is critical. Inasmuch
as a notable number of malpractice cases are tried, a successful expert must be able to command the attention and gain
the respect of the jury. You must be able to answer questions
in response to both direct and cross-examination, succinctly
and with terminology a layperson can understand. It is necessary that you be able to define terms used so that technical
concepts can be understood by the average juror. Your value

to an attorney and his client and ultimate "staying power" are determined by your capacity to communicate. If your communication skills in the lay arena are lacking, develop them.

Team Participation

Finally, you must appreciate that litigation is a team effort. Each party's attorney is charged with the responsibility of obtaining discovery, that is, information in pursuit or defense of the claims, by various means. Once discovery is complete, the lawyer then decides which witnesses will testify. In a routine malpractice matter, a party's case presentation will include testimony by that party, fact witnesses and experts. The testifying experts will be those who address the issues of liability (deviation from or compliance with the standard of care), causation (whether the criticized conduct caused or contributed to the alleged injury) and damages (the nature and extent of injury alleged to result from the defendant's conduct). In a given case, these areas of expert testimony may be addressed by one expert or multiple experts practicing in different fields. Nevertheless, the point to be remembered is that you will be but one member of the defense team, albeit a critical one. Consequently, the substance of your testimony at trial must mesh neatly with that of the other trial witnesses.

At trial, the order of witnesses will reflect the attorney's trial "design". The presentation of a party's case is determined by the attorney, who understands how to maximize the effectiveness of that presentation. As a result, you likely will be scheduled to appear in court on a day and at a time that best serves the defendant's case. Such scheduling might be less than ideal for you and your practice. However, to the extent that you are able to do so, you should be willing to adjust your professional (and certainly your personal) schedule to appear in court when it best aids the "team" and its goals. Although attorneys and, to a lesser extent, judges will try to be mindful of your practice commitments, your participation as an expert in a malpractice case necessarily requires that you recognize that you must at times endure otherwise minor scheduling inconveniences if it is in the best interest of the defendant on whose behalf you have been retained. An attorney constantly is under pressure in the preparation and presentation of the case. Members of the attorney's team who cooperate with him will be remembered—and so will those who don't. Gain a reputation as someone with whom it is easy to work.

Chapter 2

Attorney's Perspective

A valued expert in any field is one who consistently possesses qualities that render him a vital asset to the litigation team. Those qualities are multiple, and the more you have, the more you will be pursued by defense counsel in malpractice matters. Some of the assets important to the preparation and presentation of the case are more significant than others and the importance attached to each asset may vary from attorney to attorney. Suffice it to say, each is worth addressing and/or developing if you want to be considered a valued expert.

Expert Fees

In my experience, malpractice carriers and self-insured hospitals and medical centers insist on the preparation of a proper and effective defense. Yet, litigation costs can be a concern and properly so. That said, preparing both a rigorous and financially responsible defense remain parallel goals. Therefore, when you begin your expert career, your preliminary value will be measured, in part, by the cost of retaining your services. If you price yourself out of the market, little work will come your way.

Of course, you may choose to create a separate legal identity for your expert work such as an LLC. In this way, you can keep your expert service income separate from your professional practice income.

You should establish an hourly fee for document review, conferences, report preparation and deposition testimony. The prevailing hourly expert fee is in the range of $500–$750. Highly specialized or uniquely qualified individuals may enjoy hourly rates at or even above the upper end of this range. Of course, as a novice, it may be in your best interest to establish an hourly fee which is at or below the lower end of this range. If you intend to enjoy the receipt of assignments for years to come, accept the lesser rate, develop your reputation at least as an affordable expert and the rest will take care of itself. Remember that another defendant's attorney in one case may retain you as his or her expert in a different matter. If you possess the other important qualities (or most of them) that I discuss, or are capable of developing them, the hourly rates you charge and the volume of work you receive will naturally increase over time. Resist forcing the issue at the start. If your hourly rate or the time you devote to document review or to report preparation is excessive, you may be asked to curtail your effort or, worse yet, you may be infrequently retained.

You may be tempted to request a financial retainer at the outset of your expert career. Avoid the temptation. Many carriers frown at the idea of paying a retainer to an expert even one who is amply experienced. In fact, most carriers will rarely use such an expert. Certainly, as a novice expert, you should never insist on a retainer.

Be aware that the payment of an expert invoice may take some time. Upon receipt of a bill, retaining counsel must process it internally which includes following carrier/hospital guidelines for invoice transmittal and payment. Once funds for an expert invoice are received by counsel, payment is processed and a check is issued. Although you likely will receive payment within 60 days of transmittal of your invoice to counsel, there may be times when payment takes somewhat longer.

Some experts utilize a flat fee for initial document review and report preparation. This approach is generally acceptable so long as the fee (typically $2,500–$5,000) is deemed reasonable by the defense given the amount of time needed to review materials and prepare a report. A flat fee may also be charged for a deposition consuming an established maximum number of hours. This fee is paid by the plaintiff's attorney seeking the deposition, and if considered reasonable based upon the amount of time devoted to the deposition, there will be little objection. Since the precise length of a deposition usually is somewhat unpredictable, many plaintiff lawyers will not agree to a flat fee when it would result in an exorbitant financial benefit to the expert. By way of example, if the flat fee is $2,000 and the deposition ultimately consumes only two hours, such a fee results in an hourly rate of $1,000. Of course, if the deposition consumes four hours, this translates into an hourly rate of $500, which is less objectionable.

By way of further example, some experts, though not many, engage in the practice of increasing their hourly fee for depositions beyond that charged for document review and report preparation. As a result, the adverse attorney is required to pay more for the expert's time than the attorney who retained that expert. A typical explanation given is that a deposition is far more mentally taxing than document review or report preparation. Another is that document review and report preparation can be accomplished during off-hours, evenings and weekends, while a deposition is given during office hours which by definition interferes with practice time. Though this approach may seem appealing, there is a danger. Markedly increasing the hourly fee for a deposition can be used against you at trial in front of a jury. Clever adverse counsel will elicit testimony that you arbitrarily raised your hourly fee for deposition because you understood that the plaintiff's counsel (and therefore the plaintiff) was required to pay for your deposition time, thereby suggesting that you simply increased your fee to financially damage the adverse party. If your conduct can be portrayed as arbitrary, so too may your opinions.

That said, if you charge an hourly trial appearance fee that equals the hourly deposition fee, such an argument by the plaintiff's attorney is deflated. Since the defense is responsible for your trial appearance fee, you seem even-handed.

Further, you should understand that judges may become involved in establishing expert fees when necessary. As you should appreciate, billing schemes that appear to deliberately and undeservedly "squeeze" the adverse party or result in a considerable economic benefit to the expert are disfavored. If all counsel are unable to agree as to reasonable expert fees or if a party's expert demands an excessive fee, a request may be made of a judge to establish hourly rates for all experts in the matter. Although an expert is not technically bound by the court order that results from such a request, as the expert is not a party to the action, the party who is so bound and his counsel will expect the expert to accept the fee schedule established by the judge. Of course, if you choose not to (at your own peril if you are a new expert), the adverse party nevertheless will only be required to compensate you at the rate established by the court and the difference between the court-ordered rate and your rate will be borne by the party retaining you. Frankly, this is a circumstance as a new expert you should avoid. You will be perceived as overpriced at best and uncooperative at worst.

The final financial issue concerns your fee for trial testimony. Again, reasonableness is the touchstone. Trial fees, like deposition fees, can be based on an hourly rate and can include travel time. Alternatively, trial fees can be based on a flat rate. Typically, flat rates are established for either a half- or full-day appearance. Half-day fees typically range from $4,000 to $5,000 while full-day appearances are customarily charged as a flat fee of between $6,000 and $8,000. Your rate should be based on your specialty, the strength of your credentials and your experience level. As with other expert fees, attorneys (and their clients) will better respond to those perceived as appropriate and reasonable under the circum-stances. Generally, there should be no additional charges for mileage, tolls or parking expenses. However, if you are traveling out of state and are required to incur expenses such as airfare or hotel charges, it is permissible and expected that these costs will be submitted to retaining counsel for reimbursement.

Oftentimes, an expert will base his fee on lost patient billings. That is, the expert will establish a fee loosely based upon monies which otherwise would have been earned in patient billings had the expert not been in court. If, for example, a trial appearance requires the practitioner to cancel patient hours, the expert may establish an appearance fee that approximates lost patient billings. Although this approach may have some superficial appeal, its acceptability is largely dependent upon the resultant fee charged retaining counsel. If the figure falls within an acceptable range (such as that mentioned above), this method will not be criticized.

Availability

Interest alone is not enough to succeed as a malpractice defense expert. If professional and/or personal commitments unduly interfere with your service as an expert, your career will be short-lived. Availability is a multifaceted asset and remains a constant factor in an attorney's assessment of the value of an expert.

Initially, you must have sufficient available time to conduct a thorough review of the documents supplied by counsel at the time of your retention. You must also be able to com-plete that review within a reasonable period of time after receipt. Counsel will normally expect you to complete your review and issue a report in approximately three to four weeks. However, there may be occasions when unusual time constraints imposed by the court require retaining counsel to obtain the report in less than three weeks. In some jurisdictions, experts are permitted to testify at trial without the requirement that retaining counsel provide an expert report to opposing counsel in advance of trial. However, timely input from you nevertheless remains important, and the retaining attorney will certainly benefit from your review and analysis sooner rather than later. No matter the state in which the case is venued, if you can exceed expectations by completing your assignment in less time than allotted, your value is enhanced. Counsel will always appreciate such effort.

You must also be available for a deposition in those jurisdictions where they are permitted. In New Jersey, for example, an expert is routinely deposed. Although it can be scheduled in your office, an expert deposition is commonly conducted at the office of the retaining attorney. A deposition and pre-deposition meeting usually requires that you be available for three to four hours, or perhaps more. They are conducted on a business day and during normal business hours, which means that unless your deposition is scheduled on your "day off", you will be unable to schedule patients during that time. An occasional deposition may not prove to be terribly disruptive to your practice. However, as a busy expert, you may have to set time aside for depositions with some regularity. This is an obligation you cannot avoid and consequently, availability is key.

It is important to appreciate that expert depositions, like all other depositions, once scheduled are subject to adjournment by the adverse attorney. Frequently, those depositions are cancelled a day before the scheduled deposition, typically as a result of that attorney's scheduling conflicts. Should this happen, you may be tempted to charge a cancellation fee. To do so is not unreasonable, but it is essential that the existence of a cancellation fee be established at the time of retention. Retaining counsel should then advise the plaintiff's attorney of such a fee at the time your deposition is scheduled. In this way, the plaintiff's attorney cannot claim surprise and perhaps it will prevent the unnecessary "last minute" cancellation of your deposition.

Finally, you must also be available to testify at trial. Absent current COVID-19 dictated modifications, trials, like depositions, require your appearance, and like depositions, trials are conducted during the business day. As a result, you must be able to "juggle" your professional schedule so as to make yourself available when the retaining attorney deems it best. Of course, there always will be some "give and take" between defense counsel and the expert as to the date and time of a court appearance so that the expert's professional obligations are not unnecessarily disrupted or the expert unnecessarily pressured. However, if you are serious about expert work, you must be available to travel to court and participate when it might not be professionally or personally ideal to do so. As already noted, your testimony can be video-recorded prior to the trial for presentation during trial if you anticipate absolute unavailability. Most attorneys, however, consider this alternative to a live appearance less effective, and it is infrequently employed.

Accessibility

Accessibility is to be distinguished from availability. A typical malpractice case may be pending for three to five years, or longer in some jurisdictions. A defense expert likely will be contacted within the first 6–12 months of the litigation or sooner if defense counsel requires an early assessment of the liability claims, which frequently occurs. The expert will be involved for the balance of the time the matter is pending. Clearly, the expert's commitment is long term. As a result, the expert must be accessible to the retaining attorney when and if the case dictates.

A telephone or virtual conference with defense counsel in between seeing patients or at the end of your professional day may be necessary. Although defense counsel is able to discuss issues or obtain input from the defendant practitioner with relative ease, interim conferences with the retained expert will nevertheless be a critical component of the defense attorney/ defense expert relationship.

Expect there to be occasions when defense counsel or members of the attorney's staff will need to contact you to discuss matters, some mundane, some not, as the litigation proceeds. In fact, the defense of a matter might be enhanced by your participation in any number of ways. For example, you might be contacted to discuss the substance of medical records or the plaintiff's interrogatory answers or the deposition testimony obtained from a party or the plaintiff's expert as the information is gathered by counsel. On the mundane side, you may be contacted to discuss scheduling concerns, fee issues or deadline dates. No matter the issue, when the need arises to reach you, you must be reasonably accessible by telephone and/or e-mail. You must be willing to communicate with counsel or counsel's office for any number of reasons. If you have your office staff regularly run interference for you, resist getting on the phone or avoid contact with the retaining lawyer, your lack of accessibility will be duly noted, and worse, duly remembered.

Cooperation

This asset is just as much an intangible quality as it is a palpable one. Attorneys sometimes remark that an expert is "easy to work with". This is as good an expression of the concept of cooperation as any. In the context of litigation, "ease" is an elusive notion. Rarely is it part of the pressure-packed world of trial work. Yet, if it can be found even in small doses, it is treasured—and it is not forgotten.

In general terms, a cooperative expert is one who reflects the best of the first three values already mentioned. Reasonable fees, availability and accessibility, as explained above, combine to define an expert who is "easy to work with". Of course, there are degrees of cooperation, and professional and/or personal obligations may render you more or less cooperative during your work on a given case. Reputation as a cooperative member of the litigation team cannot be underestimated. Frankly, it is one of the qualities that I find myself and other attorneys often discussing when selecting an expert in a given discipline. Ultimately, cooperation without other qualities will not itself make you a valued expert. But, it's a great start.

Credentials

Before a jury ever hears you utter a word about your opinions, it will hear about your credentials. Similarly, before you ever get a chance to impress a retaining attorney with your thinking about an issue, that attorney likely will consider the appropriateness of retaining you based on an understanding of your background. Indeed, your credentials will determine whether defense counsel even contacts you. It is essential, therefore, that you prepare a compelling Curriculum Vitae (CV).

Your CV should be in a form that is easily read and understood. Later, I will discuss in detail the creation of an effective CV. For now, simply remember that the CV in this context is a marketing tool. It should be designed as such. The print should be large and legible. Resist using a fancy font style or small font. A document that can be reviewed with ease (there's that treasured concept again) will be favorably received.

Enough said about form. Let's address substance. Before you are permitted to offer testimony in court, the trial judge must "qualify" you as an expert. That is, the judge must make a preliminary determination as to whether you should be allowed to offer opinions to the jury.

Non-expert or fact witnesses do not have to be "qualified" by the court as they are not typically asked (or permitted) to offer their opinions. In a malpractice case, for example, the plaintiff will testify about the condition that prompted treatment from the defendant practitioner, the treatment obtained, his or her current condition and the limitations imposed by that condition. The defendant also will offer testimony about the relevant facts. Perhaps other treaters will testify, as might members of the plaintiff's family, friends or co-workers. The testimony offered by such individuals is factual in nature and commonly focuses only on what was done, seen, heard, said or thought. With rare legal exception, fact witnesses do not offer their opinions.

Experts, however, do provide opinion testimony. Indeed, that is their role. Although they will offer testimony about the facts, as they understand them, such comment serves only as a prelude to the opinions that must be based on those facts. (To the extent that the expert's understanding of the facts is erroneous, the opinions based on such errant information will be compromised and be of little ultimate value to the jury who must assess their worth.)

In a manner of speaking, the judge is the "gatekeeper" charged with the responsibility of ensuring that the jury receives opinion testimony only from those who are "competent" to give it. Consequently, unlike fact witnesses who typically are not called upon to furnish opinions, a proposed expert must provide testimony about his or her education, training and experience so that the judge may assess the propriety of allowing that witness to offer opinion testimony.

As a general proposition, judges will permit a witness to testify as an expert with little more than the minimal requirements established by individual state law. Such basic qualifications, however, do little to enhance an expert's value before a jury or further the cause of the litigant on whose behalf the expert has been retained. Unlike judges, who simply seek to ensure that the offered expert is "competent" to testify, attorneys typically strive to retain the "ideal" expert for a case. That assessment in the first instance is based on the expert's credentials. Although a professional license may suffice as a minimum predicate to testifying as an expert in many jurisdictions, state law may require actual practice experience by those who serve as experts. Moreover, defense attorneys will not be comfortable presenting a novice practitioner as an expert at trial. Convincing a jury of the legitimacy of an expert's opinion is difficult. If that expert is relatively inexperienced, an otherwise daunting task becomes almost impossible. Consequently, if you have been in practice for a very short time, it is doubtful that you will be able to attract much expert work. An attorney seeking an expert will likely pass on most individuals who do not have at least ten years of experience in the field. Of course, there may be exceptions, but they are likely to be few and far between. In my opinion, at the ten-year mark, a practitioner has an experience base sufficient to offer meaningful comment in most instances. More important, with at least ten years of experience, an expert's opinions will not be questioned by the jury simply because of perceived inexperience. Frankly, my comfort level with an expert increases exponentially with the number of years my expert has been in practice. I suspect that juries react the same way.

Understand that trial counsel will seize any opportunity to undermine the opinions of the adverse expert. If the expert is truly inexperienced or if the expert can be portrayed as relatively inexperienced (when compared to the opposing expert), a threshold issue can be created which will swing the pendulum of courtroom advantage in favor of the party who has exposed the adverse expert as a novice practitioner.

Of course, there comes a point at which an expert's wealth of experience becomes a liability. Although a senior member of the profession typically is a welcome addition to the defense team, a jury's reaction to such an individual may not always be as positive as one might expect. Experts who have "slowed down", that is, those who have reduced their patient load, stopped performing certain procedures, partially retired or relinquished part of their practice to younger colleagues have limited value as liability experts in malpractice cases. The exception is that individual recognized in the field as "the authority" on a subject or whose experience base is so overwhelmingly superior to that of the average practitioner that his or her senior status is more of an advantage than a disadvantage. Apart from such an exceptional case, however, it is a sure bet that opposing counsel at trial will exploit the expert's vulnerability on this level.

In addition to looking for an expert with the requisite years of experience and who practices in the specialty of the defendant, defense counsel also will want an expert who is board certified in that field (if certification is available). Since the public is acutely aware of the significance of board certification, this credential is important to possess.

If becoming board certified required multiple attempts, disclose this information to retaining counsel at the time retention is discussed. Although failed attempts are unfortunate, oftentimes legitimate reasons exist for their occurrence.

Since the board-certified practitioner is generally viewed by the lay individual as superior to the uncertified one, the successful satisfaction of all certification requirements is perceived as an impressive accomplishment. It is for that reason that most skilled malpractice attorneys will ask the retained expert at trial to describe the certification regimen in some detail. Without question, jurors are receptive both to the testimony about the board certification process and, in most instances, the expert who successfully completes it. If you are not yet board certified, get board certified. If you choose not to, in all likelihood, you will never be retained by malpractice counsel as an expert.

Other important credentials which have value to the retaining lawyer include graduation from prestigious American universities, medical schools or osteopathic schools, internship and residency programs, fellowship programs, privileges (ranging from full attending to courtesy) at area medical centers and hospitals, academic positions in professional schools, membership in medical societies and specialty organizations, professional awards and honors, publications, presentations, lectures and seminars, just to name a few. Although attendance at a foreign medical school can be less impressive than attendance at an American institution, it will not preclude you from expert service. The circumstances may be such that attending a foreign school could prove beneficial and not necessarily detrimental.

To the extent that your CV includes many, if not most, of these, all the better. The absence of any one (or more) of them, however, should not serve to discourage you, as your worth as an expert derives from consideration of numerous factors. Alternatively, the more impressive your CV is, the more encouraging are your prospects of becoming a defense expert. If attaining additional credentials is possible, I urge you to give careful thought to doing so. Not only will counsel's (and more important, a jury's) perception of you be positively affected, your stature among your colleagues and your patients also will be boosted. Indeed, I think it fair to say that anything you do in the name of becoming a more attractive malpractice expert will have the added bonus of benefitting you on a number of professional levels outside the world of malpractice litigation.

Reasonable Standards

As you must appreciate, the reason a liability defense expert is contacted in most instances is to lend assistance to the successful defense of a pending lawsuit. This can only be accomplished if the expert is in a position to know the applicable standard of care. Deviation from the accepted standard of care is a common legal definition of the term "malpractice", which may also be called "professional negligence". The standard of care is generally defined as that conduct which is considered acceptable under the given circumstances by members of the profession. Malpractice, therefore, may result from a departure from the standard of care in the performance of an act or in the failure to act. It may also arise in that instance where a practitioner does not obtain a patient's informed consent to treatment, that is, fails to disclose all of the material risks associated with such treatment, the benefits and the reasonable alternatives.

The ability to apply a standard of care to a set of facts presupposes knowledge of that standard. Knowledge of a standard of care presumes that the expert is in a position to know. Although this seems elementary, it may be overlooked. Be mindful that without an appropriate knowledge base, your value as an expert is reduced if not eliminated.

By way of example, some years ago I tried a malpractice case on behalf of a podiatrist who was alleged to have negligently performed surgery on the plaintiff. Many months prior to the trial, I received a copy of the liability report and CV of the plaintiff's rather young podiatry expert. Thereafter, the plaintiff's expert testified at deposition that he was attending podiatry school at the time my client performed the subject surgery. During my cross-examination of the expert at trial, I again elicited testimony from him that on the date my client had performed the criticized surgery, the plaintiff's expert was a student. Without ever having performed the type of procedure in the manner it was typically performed during the years he was a student, the witness conceded that he had no real knowledge of the practical application of the standard of care to the subject facts. Armed with that testimony,

I suspended my cross-examination of the expert, asked the court to temporarily excuse the jury from the courtroom and argued for dismissal of the Complaint. Without an expert to testify as to the manner in which the standard of care applied to my client's conduct, the plaintiff could not offer proof about any alleged deviation from the applicable standard. As a result, the plaintiff's case was fatally flawed. The trial judge retired to his chambers to consider my application and returned with the pronouncement my client and I both wanted to hear— Complaint dismissed.

Clearly, it is not enough for you as a potential liability expert to be able to identify the standard of care. If that were sufficient, my podiatry case would have concluded with a jury verdict rather than a court-ordered dismissal. Certainly, in that example, the plaintiff's expert, a practicing podiatrist at the time he authored his report, was capable of identifying a standard of care. After all, he read about the subject procedure while a podiatry student. Reading about something, however, may not give you a base of practical knowledge upon which to draw. Had the plaintiff's expert testified that he had knowledge of the manner in which the standard of care applied to my client's performance of the surgery, even though he had never performed the procedure, he would have been permitted to offer an opinion about the standard and the manner in which my client deviated from it. The expert's lack of practical experience would simply have affected his credibility, that is, the weight the jury might have given to his testimony. It would not in itself have deprived the plaintiff of the opportunity to have a jury resolve the parties' dispute. The witness, however, honestly testified that given his lack of experience with the procedure, he did not know the standard's practical application to the subject circumstances. It was that truthful testimony which caused the trial judge to dismiss the matter.

I should add that some weeks after the conclusion of the trial, I received a telephone call from an attorney who had been retained by that plaintiff to investigate the conduct of the plaintiff's lawyer as related to the retention of the plaintiff's expert. Apparently, consideration was being given to filing a legal malpractice case against that attorney for having retained an inappropriate expert. The theory was that the retaining counsel should have obtained the services of a liability expert who had sufficient experience to know how the standard of care applied to my client. Suffice it to say, this was an interesting twist to what appeared to be a straightforward malpractice case when it first came into my firm.

Without question, if you intend to offer your services as a liability expert, you must understand the term "minimal standards". This concept is best defined as conduct that minimally comports with professionally appropriate behavior. You must also be familiar with the term "optimal standards". This concept perhaps is best defined as conduct that exceeds minimal standards and reflects behavior that ideally suits the circumstances. Typically, most professionals practice somewhere between minimal standards and optimal standards.

As an expert, you must be able to recognize gradations of appropriate behavior and, of course, you must be able to identify behavior that falls below minimal standards. Keep in mind that as a liability expert you are expected to know and be able to discuss the standard of care that governs a defendant's conduct. The standard of care may be absolutely consistent with that which you would do under similar circumstances or it may be different.

For example, different treatment options in a given circumstance might all satisfy the standard of care. Because your treatment recommendation might differ from that of a defendant does not mean that the practitioner has deviated from the standard of care so long as such recommendation has support in the profession as appropriate under the circumstances. By way of further example, you may take action in a certain situation that equals or even exceeds optimal standards. The defendant, however, need not meet your individual standard of care in order to satisfy the standard of care that generally applies to the situation. You must be able to assess the defendant's conduct in the context of that which is generally expected of the practitioner, not what you necessarily would do under similar circumstances.

That said, if your individual practice standards in a given situation exceed those followed by the defendant, such disparity likely will be exposed by adverse counsel at trial to the detriment of the defense. Therefore, it is essential that you disclose this fact to the retaining attorney as early as possible so that defense counsel can determine whether you are the appropriate defense expert.

The retaining attorney needs the assistance of a liability expert who is capable of identifying reasonable standards that govern a defendant's actions. Just as a plaintiff's expert might use inappropriately strict standards so as to conclude that a defendant's actions deviated from the standard of care, you may be tempted to endorse liberal standards in the interest of defense service. Resist the temptation and exercise caution. Although you may be well intentioned, never endorse standards that are too lax. Ultimately, you do a disservice to the defense (and yourself) if you identify a standard of care that is designed solely to exculpate the defendant without regard to accepted practice. A defense expert who is too liberal will be exposed under effective cross-examination by a skilled plaintiff's attorney. As a result, the opinions of such a defense expert will be rejected by the jury when weighed against the more reasonable opinions of the adverse expert.

Indeed, attorneys seeking expert opinions assume you will offer reasonable ones. With that in mind, the successful defense of a malpractice matter absolutely requires your candid assessment. If you aspire to become a credible expert, focus on establishing yourself as one who employs and applies consistently reasonable standards. In the long run, you will be respected and appreciated by the defense bar for doing so.

Report Preparation

Although the liability expert report will be discussed later in greater detail, some brief remarks are warranted here. Suffice it to say, where required by a particular jurisdiction and/ or requested by retaining counsel, the liability report of the expert witness typically is critical. Without question, there is no substitute for a well-thought-out and a well-written expert report. Certainly, your worth as an expert initially will be judged by the report you generate. It typically is the "jewel" of the case in that it crystallizes the essence of the defense and is the best expression of the matter from the perspective of the defendant on whose behalf the report has been written. The liability expert report is more powerful than any argument that might be prepared by an attorney concerning the substantive issues in the case simply because it is written by someone who has the credentials to know about the issues addressed. Indeed, it is a precursor to what the jury will ultimately hear (and hopefully accept).

The liability expert report also gains its importance from the fact that well before a jury learns its content, the attorney retaining you does. Although it is likely that you have discussed your thoughts with the retaining lawyer before preparing your report, seeing those thoughts in writing is satisfying to counsel. The impact of the expert report on the retaining lawyer cannot be overestimated. The report lends a certain degree of tangible legitimacy to what were previously conceptual defenses. It represents the very foundation upon which all else will be built. Of course, if the report is served on adverse counsel, as is required in certain states, it has the further effect of alerting opposing counsel (and the plaintiff) of the merit to the defenses being raised. The stronger the report, the greater the impact. It also may prove beneficial in connection with settlement negotiations, mediation or arbitration if settlement is contemplated.

Given the multifaceted significance of the liability expert report and given the fact that the report is an expression of your assessment of the case, significant effort must be devoted to its preparation. The report must reflect your best thinking about the issues and that thinking must be presented in an organized and understandable fashion. In sum, the report must be a document that you are proud to author and that the retaining attorney is proud to utilize.

Insulation from Collateral Examination

A well-insulated expert is a desirable one. No attorney knowingly retains a liability expert who is easily subject to "collateral attack". This term describes attorney examination that elicits information about the expert that adversely affects the expert's credibility, even though it might be irrelevant to the substantive issues in the case. Understand that an expert may offer substantive testimony at trial that appears to be incredible when tested by effective cross-examination or when contradicted by the more reasoned and/or reasonable testimony of the adverse expert. Such attacks are commonplace. Further, since the parties' liability experts typically disagree about the pivotal issues at trial, resolution of those issues necessarily means that juries must reject (in whole or in part) the testimony of someone's expert. Attorneys understand and accept that this is the process. Of course, as the trial progresses, it is the lawyer's expectation that the case will be developed in such a way that ultimately his expert and, therefore, his client will prevail.

Attacks on experts at trial that are collateral to the merits of the case, but that test an expert's credibility, can be effective, perhaps more so than attempts to discredit an expert's substantive opinions. The subjects of such examination are too numerous to list. However, a few examples will illustrate the point:

1. Limited clinical experience (due to any number of reasons, including semi-retirement, reduction in patient numbers, elimination of certain practice procedures or academic and/or administrative responsibilities);
2. The absence of publications regarding the issues raised by the lawsuit;
3. The absence of invitations to speak nationally and/or internationally;
4. The absence of formal presentations or lectures regarding the the issues raised by the lawsuit; and
5. The absence of any formal academic position.

These are but a few of the collateral matters that can create a problem. As you can see, you may be subject to collateral examination in one case and yet be insulated from such examination in another case. Attorneys are always concerned about retaining experts who are subject to this type of attack. Trials are difficult enough to win without having to worry about an expert who, before addressing the substance of the case, is capable of being neutralized by collateral issues.

Consequently, it is important that you candidly advise retaining counsel about your credentials and experience. The complete disclosure of information relevant to such possible examination at the time of retention is critical. Avoid accepting assignments where your participation may hurt the case more than help it. Remember, counsel is charged with the responsibility of presenting the best possible defense at trial. To that end, trial witnesses retained to enhance that effort must be insulated from significant collateral examination.

Although of minimal concern at the start of your expert career, as that career expands, you must be diligent about disclosing to retaining counsel your involvement in other similar cases where your opinions do not support the defense theory in the new matter. Of course, every malpractice case is unique. However, there may well be an identity of issues between the new matter and other matters in which you have participated. Assume that the plaintiff's bar has access to your previously expressed opinions and will use them in cross-examination if the circumstances warrant. Consequently, disclosure is essential. "Surprise" testimony about inconsistent prior opinions will serve to damage the defense at the worst possible time—at trial. Accordingly, counsel will expect a reasonable degree of consistency from case to case in the opinions you offer, and any variation (no matter the reason) must be revealed as early as possible.

It also is worth noting that as you attract more work, the percentage of annual income earned from expert work may become the focus of a collateral attack. The greater the percentage over time, the more likely adverse counsel will exploit that fact.

Handling Examination

Descriptions such as "good in court", "trial savvy" and "an experienced witness" are all used by malpractice attorneys to identify an expert who is a capable witness. Such an expert can respond to both direct and cross-examination effectively. The importance of the qualities thus far discussed, which might otherwise help to make you a valued expert, pales in comparison to your ability to capably answer questions posed in the courtroom. If you can articulately and convincingly respond to examination by attorneys in what most likely will be an unfamiliar environment (at least in the early years of your expert career) without faltering, you will survive and indeed thrive as a malpractice expert.

The ability to effectively communicate your opinions before a jury requires an understanding of the examination process. Although you may have experience speaking at seminars or teaching in classrooms, with some exceptions, courtroom testimony is not akin to lecturing colleagues or instructing residents. The most obvious difference stems from the manner in which you are permitted to comment in court: that is, by responding to questions. You must also understand that unlike speaking engagements of the type mentioned above, as a trial witness, you have only limited control over the manner in which you present the subject matter.

Assuming you have reviewed the scope and substance of your anticipated testimony with the retaining attorney before your court appearance (which is essential to an effective presentation), you will know the areas that will be the focus of direct examination by that attorney, and the attorney should know what you will say in response. Of course, retaining counsel will ultimately determine the direction of your direct testimony. Remain true to your preparation and always resist throwing a "curve ball" to retaining counsel at trial by providing unanticipated testimony about unimportant matters or by simply offering an opinion never before disclosed to that attorney.

There likely will be occasions when a question posed by the retaining attorney will naturally require a somewhat lengthy and detailed response. Your answer may be enhanced by the use of trial exhibits, perhaps anatomical models, displays, drawings or PowerPoint images requiring that you leave the witness stand and position yourself directly in front of the jury box, when testifying live. These opportunities are golden, and it is in this circumstance where you will likely be able to conduct a mini lecture and direct its content (with the caveat that the "presentation" is responsive to the question posed). When this occurs, it is crucial that you grab the jury's attention and hold on to it. At no other time during your testimony will you be in such control of the courtroom, and you must take advantage of the moment.

Effective testimony in response to examination by the retaining attorney requires that you answer questions posed in a concise, understandable and precise manner. Let me explain.

A concise response is a brief one. No one wants to listen to a ten-minute diatribe when a ten-word answer will suffice. It is important to understand that the attention span of most people is limited and, given the fact that trials are time-consuming, your effectiveness in significant part depends on your ability to "reach" the jury. If your answers are unnecessarily long and your testimony tedious as a result, you will likely cause jurors to "shut down". Once that happens, little you say will be absorbed. The sound of your voice, no matter how intriguing to you, will simply become background noise as your opinions bounce off the jury like so many ping pong balls at a table tennis tournament. A carefully constructed, crisp presentation with an economy of words is key. You must keep the jurors interested in your opinions by not boring them with too much verbiage.

Your answers also must be understandable. Of course, it is essential that an expert witness impress the jury as an authority in his or her field. Facility with the subject matter and the technical terminology must be demonstrated. However, jurors are lay individuals and generally lack familiarity with technical concepts and terminology. Consequently, explanations of principles and professional terms must be included in your direct testimony. Although examining counsel should and likely will ask you to define technical terms you reference, voluntary explanations of strange terminology by you in the course of an answer will be much appreciated by the jury as reflected in the occasional head nod.

Finally, a precise answer is one that addresses the question presented. It avoids superfluous preludes or explanations. It focuses on the heart of the question and prompts a sense of satisfaction in the listener because the question has been addressed by the substance of the response. Simply stated, a precise answer "cuts to the chase".

In addition to providing an adequate explanation of the technical components of a given case, discuss their application to the facts in a way that is clear. Jurors are generally capable of thinking logically about the issues presented. In order to aid them in that process, it is crucial that your testimony make sense. No matter how brilliant you are or how thick your CV is, if you are difficult to follow, you and your opinions will be rejected. As trial attorneys, we expect orderly, organized and understandable testimony from our experts. Circuitous reasoning and technical "mumbo-jumbo" serve no purpose in court.

All of the requirements discussed above which make for effective direct testimony also apply to an expert's answers to cross-examination. The obvious difference is that the retaining lawyer conducts direct examination while adverse counsel conducts cross-examination. This difference is important because direct questions must be couched in an open-ended fashion allowing you, in fact, requiring you to provide substantive responses. Cross-examination, however, is typically self-limiting. That is, such questions are usually leading in nature and most often seek only a "yes" or "no" answer. Consequently, you will have little opportunity to dazzle or impress. On those rare occasions where you are given that chance, take advantage of it. Remember again, however, to be concise, understandable and precise.

Cross-examination requires that you be able to "think on your feet". You must be sufficiently facile with concepts applicable to your practice area and with the obvious and at times less obvious factual details of the case to capably respond to the questions posed. Of course, you must also be aware of the strengths and weaknesses of the defense you are assisting as well as the theories supporting that defense. In this way, you will ensure (to the extent possible) that your testimony will mesh with and not run counter to such theories. At all times, you must have your wits about you so as to avoid even an inadvertent statement that might do damage. However, should it be necessary, retaining counsel can always conduct redirect examination to address damaging remarks made or weaknesses exposed during cross-examination.

In the end, if you remain true to the principles on which your opinions are based, you likely will successfully withstand even fierce cross-examination by the most skilled attorneys. Always remember, a typical malpractice lawyer, no matter how competent, does not have the technical education and training possessed by the expert. Consequently, in a difficult spot during cross-examination, reliance on what you know as a practitioner should place you in a superior position and allow you to win the battle with adverse counsel.

There is no substitute for an expert who is capable of effectively functioning as a courtroom witness. Testimony both in response to direct and cross-examination supplied in a manner consistent with the above precepts is invaluable. If you are capable of becoming such a witness, you will prove to be a formidable member of the defense team and your reputation will be enhanced.

Credibility

Credibility is a vague, somewhat amorphous concept that is not easily defined in this context. Yet it is a quality essential to your success as an expert. Not only must the substance of your testimony be credible, you must also appear to be a credible individual. Indeed, a jury will more readily accept the opinions of a witness if that witness' testimony is cloaked with a veil of believability. Some people just seem to have a credible air about them. Perhaps it's a manner of speech, a sincere appearance or a confident personality. Such individuals draw people in and are more capable than others of easily convincing total strangers of the wisdom of their thinking. Their ability to appear credible may be an inherent quality requiring little work. Those who don't have this "gift" may nevertheless prove to be credible trial witnesses. It may simply require more effort. With such individuals, this "acquired" credibility, however, will stem more from the substance of the expert's testimony than simply from the witness' courtroom demeanor.

In either circumstance, unless a jury is convinced that you are credible, your opinions will be rejected. This eventuality can be ill afforded by counsel and client given that liability expert testimony typically is the cornerstone of any malpractice action. If the expert falters, in most instances, so too will the defense.

Consequently, attorneys always seek to retain credible experts. If you're convinced of the legitimacy of the litigant's position, it is likely that your ability to deliver credible testimony in court will be enhanced. Simply stated, if you don't "buy" it, you will have a difficult time trying to "sell" it to a group of jurors. The jury will "size you up" during your testimony, and if you appear insincere, the jury will be more likely to reject your opinions. Resist the temptation to accept an assignment where to do so requires you to compromise yourself. If you are unable to offer legitimate expert opinion in defense of a malpractice claim, walk away. Otherwise, you likely will have a difficult time in court appearing credible. Conversely, if you can legitimately support the defendant practitioner and can do so vigorously, your courtroom testimony naturally will have a sense of credibility about it that will serve to enhance the likelihood of ultimate success.

Personality

Just as people are drawn to those whose personality compels acceptance outside the courtroom, jurors are more likely to listen approvingly to a witness, expert or otherwise, whose personality enhances that witness' testimony. This quality is not something that is easily defined. An expert who attracts those around him just by virtue of his personality is a rare commodity. Of course, the substance of the expert's testimony is always more important than mere form. However, an expert who offers opinions that are substantively persuasive and who does so with pizzazz will likely prevail over an expert whose testimony, though logical, is lifeless.

If you are interested in expert work and doubt that you have the personality for courtroom performance, think again. Trial testimony is neither a "stand-up routine" nor a vaudeville act. It is not great drama, although it can be rather dramatic. By personality, I mean to convey the importance of testifying in a manner that invites—no, demands—attention. Although someone who by virtue of a gregarious personality may have an advantage over someone who is less extroverted at a cocktail party, the personality of which I speak is more complex a concept. Indeed, it is difficult to precisely describe or define the type of personality ideally suited to expert work. Perhaps, the term charisma is a good start. But use of this term has its limitations in this context as well.

There certainly are individuals whose personalities are not well suited to serving as courtroom experts. Though they may be bright and accomplished and able to craft sterling expert reports, they may simply lack the ability to project positively in a public forum. It is likely that most of you don't fall into this category. Even if you are the retiring type, a solid trial personality can be developed over time. Indeed, service as a trial witness itself will afford you the opportunity to learn what works and what doesn't. Gauging the response of jurors to your presentation is one way to determine the effectiveness of your courtroom personality and whether to make adjustments to your trial "persona". Of course, the retaining attorney is certainly an excellent resource in this regard. After all, the lawyer who hired you has a vested interest in ensuring your success. In fact, if retaining counsel likes enough things about you to consider retaining you again, it is in counsel's interest, and that of the next client, to offer constructive criticism.

That having been said, I am not suggesting that you be "reinvented". But if you are serious about serving as a malpractice expert and are interested in enhancing your value to attorneys who might seek your services, try to develop the personality that may lie just beneath the surface. It can be done.

I'm reminded of heavyweight fighter George Foreman. In his boxing heyday, I dare say that few knew that Mr. Foreman had the engaging personality he has displayed in more recent years. A warm, inviting and less imposing individual emerged. As a result, George Foreman has become a product "pitch man" convincing the public at large to purchase the goods and services he endorses. Without question, his success outside the boxing ring is directly related to his personality. Need I say more?

Attorneys looking for a "pitch man" in the malpractice arena also will fix on someone who can do for their clients what George Foreman has done for various products—sell them. Without being overly simplistic, the job of the expert is to convince total strangers to accept what the litigant is offering. You must understand this. You must also appreciate what lawyers already know: A winning personality is just that—a winning personality.

Appearance

Last, but not necessarily least, on the list of qualities that attorneys seek in a malpractice expert is best described as appearance. Although the "right look" is important, I will not suggest that this factor is overwhelmingly critical. However, there indeed are practitioners whose appearance will serve to enhance that witness' courtroom presentation.

Of course, at a minimum it is expected that you dress appropriately. Men should wear a dark suit, preferably navy blue, gray, black or brown. Avoid wearing light-colored suits. Generally speaking, do not wear casual clothing. Of course, if the trial is located in a rural area, a sports jacket may be an acceptable alternative. Otherwise, you should not wear blazers. Sweaters or vests without a suit jacket are not acceptable. This is a trial, not a golf outing. Your dress shirt should be white or light blue. Always wear a conservative tie and avoid wearing jewelry other than a watch and a wedding ring. Wear dress shoes and socks—no casual footgear.

In a recent summertime trial, my experienced expert appeared in court to testify wearing a blazer and slacks, a casual shirt (with a tie thankfully) and pastel-colored canvas slip-ons without socks. I was told it was his day off. Perhaps, this explained his relaxed attire—perhaps not. Suffice it to say, no explanation can excuse the inexcusable.

Women should abide by the recommendations above as they relate to the color of suits selected. Although professional dresses are acceptable, I prefer that women wear suits. Of course, patterned blouses should be subdued. Shoes should be conservative and dark in color. A woman can wear some jewelry but again the "look" should be understated. In sum, your attire like your purpose should be anything but frivolous.

If you wear glasses, terrific. If you have reading glasses, bring them to the witness stand and use them. In my judgment, glasses serve to make you appear more professorial and since academicians are generally respected, this look is a positive.

Excessively long hair and untrimmed beards on a man generally are detractions and should be avoided. Women should wear their hair in a businesslike fashion. Hairstyles will obviously reflect individual preferences but generally should always reflect a professional personality.

I am a strong believer in the power of nonverbal communication. From the moment I see the jury panel (prospective jurors from whom the jury for a given trial will be selected), I am watching them. I am studying their faces. I am interpreting their body language. I am examining their clothing. From this group will be selected the jury which will decide the fate of my client. It is important, therefore, that I learn as much as possible even before a prospective juror utters a word. By the time the jurors are placed in the jury box, each one will have made an initial nonverbal impression on me. It may be generally positive or it may be generally negative.

It is no different with an expert. When your name is called as the next witness and you make your way to the witness stand, you are being watched by the jury. By the time you are seated, most of the jurors will already have formed an impression of you. What do they say about first impressions?

The importance of the jury's impression of an expert based on appearance should not be ignored. As an expert you want to make sure that to the extent you can influence that impression simply by your appearance, do so. The retaining attorney will expect you to make every effort to promote an appropriate image.

Chapter 3

Jury's Perspective

Having reviewed those qualities that will make you a welcome addition to any defense team and therefore someone who attorneys will retain, you must also appreciate that to the extent your service will include trial testimony, there are certain individual qualities to which juries respond and which therefore are worth discussing. Some of what I address below may overlap values already reviewed. To the extent that occurs, the importance of those qualities cannot be overstated. Indeed, a significant percentage of malpractice lawsuits are resolved by trial. Consequently, a malpractice expert should expect to appear before a jury, rendering the following discussion extremely relevant.

Presentation

Preparation, preparation, preparation. Without question, an effective presentation at trial requires effective preparation before trial. Although this may seem all too obvious and perhaps terribly simplistic, the importance of preparation cannot be stressed enough. That you previously reviewed

the materials after agreeing to serve as a liability expert does
not mean you are prepared to testify in court. That you once
understood the details of the case doesn't mean you still
understand them months if not years later. That you authored
a well-crafted expert report doesn't mean that you are ready to
appear before a jury. The point to be made is that the presentation of your testimony requires preparation.

Typically, retaining counsel will review the matter with
you prior to your court appearance. This might occur weeks
but more likely days before you are scheduled to appear in
court. Meaningful participation in such a conference with
counsel requires that you devote the time necessary, usually significant hours, before that meeting, reacquainting
yourself with the subject matter. If you are able to discuss
the obscure details of the case with the retaining attorney
just prior to trial, it is likely that you will be able to do so in
court. That does not mean that you should not again conduct
a review on your own the day or evening before your actual
appearance—you should. Of course, if the facts are somewhat complex, more time must be devoted to your preparation. If the facts are relatively uncomplicated, less time will
be required. Either way, however, the key is time. It must
be invested in preparation before you step foot inside the
courtroom. If your preparation is lacking so too will be your
presentation. Not only will retaining counsel recognize your
failure to adequately prepare, so too will opposing counsel.
If that occurs, the adverse attorney, sensing your vulnerability,
will do everything possible to exploit your lack of familiarity
with the details of the case. Your "stock" as an expert at
trial will drop precipitously from the jury's perspective, and as
a result, the jurors will likely reject your opinions in whole or
in significant part.

If you cannot or will not devote the time necessary to
adequately prepare for your testimony, it matters little that you
authored a fabulous expert report, or that you gave compelling

deposition testimony. In the end, the trial is what matters and your presentation at trial must be convincing. If you've done your homework, the likelihood is that you'll capably handle direct and cross-examination. If you haven't, you will be ineffective at best and embarrassed at worst.

Organization

Once you have mentally prepared for courtroom testimony, it is important that you do so physically. Chances are the case in which you are involved has itself generated a fair amount of review material. As discussed in prior sections, the documents supplied to you for consideration during the course of the litigation likely have included volumes of patient records, interrogatory answers and deposition transcripts. It is also likely that the documents forwarded to you have not been received all at one time. Probably, an initial package of material was supplied at the time of your retention and supplemental transmittals were sent intermittently thereafter. As a result, documents were reviewed by you at various points in time, multiple reports were prepared (if required) and the materials were not reviewed again unless absolutely necessary.

After "dusting off" the documents and discussing the case with retaining counsel, you may be asked to bring your file to court. Of course, if the file is on a thumb drive, a disc or stored electronically in your laptop, you can bring them to court, if retaining counsel asks you to do so.

In my view, the whole point of having your file in court is two-pronged. When adverse counsel on cross-examination asks if you brought your file with you, the better answer is always "yes". Appearing with your file is more impressive than appearing without it. Additionally, although documents marked as trial exhibits by counsel will be available to you, not all of the materials you reviewed will have been so marked. As a result, should questioning make it necessary to reference a document not marked as a trial exhibit, you will benefit from having that document with you, electronically or otherwise. Adverse counsel may choose to not have you search your file for the document. But the fact that you can readily locate it and are willing to do so, may be enough to convince the jury that you have the information referenced during your direct testimony.

This having been said, it naturally follows that effective use of your file requires some form of organization. If your file is electronic, the issue of organization is less concerning. However, if your file is in paper form, trucking voluminous documents into the courtroom is only half the battle. The other half is document management. If your file is disorganized, so too may be your answers to questions that require reference to a discrete portion of that file. Over the years, I have enjoyed watching opposing experts squirm on the stand during cross-examination as they rifle through their file in an effort to locate the source of a point made during direct testimony. Although confident in a recalled fact, when asked to locate the document in which the information appears, an otherwise capable adverse expert looks downright incompetent when unable to find the supporting document. That is not to say that the document doesn't exist or that the expert has fabricated the fact. In all likelihood, the opposite is true. But if the expert is unable to find the item, the damage has been done. The jury will think the testimony of the expert is based on sheer fantasy. Again, mission accomplished.

To avoid this pitfall, it is strongly recommended that you organize the paper or electronic file before your court appearance. Use any system with which you're comfortable. With a paper file, binders with dividers and tabs that identify the material in each section is recommended. One binder may contain the plaintiff's discovery, such as interrogatory answers and deposition transcripts. A second binder may contain similar material produced on behalf of my client. Additional binders may contain the plaintiff's medical records.

Of course, it matters not the type of system you select. But you must have a system that maximizes your effectiveness in court. A disorganized expert runs the risk of being exposed as such, and frankly, this is a risk you need not take.

Subject Familiarity

After you have properly prepared for a courtroom appearance and have organized the file for ease of access, effective testimony requires that you demonstrate familiarity with the subject matter of the case. Not only must you appear facile in your ability to discuss the substantive area of practice but you also must be able to handily discuss the facts. If you have devoted adequate time to a review of the pertinent documents and to development of a system of document organization, you should be able to answer questions by counsel in a manner that reflects your effort. This is key.

Once you have been qualified by the trial judge as an expert and therefore allowed to offer opinion testimony, it is natural for the jury to expect you to "sound" like an expert. As such, your role is to aid the jury in its effort to appreciate the substantive issues, the relevant facts and the standard of care. To that end, it is essential that the jury accept your testimony. Accomplishment of this goal necessarily requires that you appear (and therefore be) conversant with the subject matter of the case. Simply stated, if you seem to know what you're talking about, the jury likely will be more accepting of what you have to say. Your effectiveness as a trial witness is supported by the ability to convey to the jurors that you are sufficiently familiar with the case to render your testimony worthy of belief. If you are deficient in this regard, and as a result are forced to "fudge", meander, avoid or concoct in response to certain questions posed, expect the jury (with the aid of opposing counsel) to reject your answers—and perhaps the rest of your testimony in the process.

Question Responsiveness

A first cousin of subject familiarity is "question responsiveness". Answering questions in a direct fashion suggests forthrightness and enhances credibility. Although this should be easily accomplished when responding to direct examination (if you and defense counsel have prepared properly), it is less so when dealing with cross-examination by adverse counsel. There is a real temptation to return to and reiterate "themes" of the case when answering questions which tangentially relate to one of those "themes". This temptation must be recognized and avoided. Although you may see merit to injecting matters into your answer extraneous to the pending question so as to refocus the jury's attention on something important to your opinion or your perspective of the facts, to do so invariably is a mistake. To do so repeatedly is a big mistake. Inevitably, one or more of the following will occur: (1) The questioning attorney will ask you to answer the question posed, suggesting that you have deliberately avoided the question; (2) the questioning attorney will ask that the trial judge direct you to answer the question posed; (3) the questioning attorney will ask that the trial judge strike your answer as not responsive and instruct the jury to disregard it or (4) the trial judge will admonish you to listen to the question and answer what's being asked. If this happens often enough, the jury will quickly conclude that you are intent on avoiding the questions posed. You may appear arrogant, sneaky or both. Ultimately, you will be perceived as an unduly evasive "advocate" with an agenda (which you are not) rather than a neutral independent expert (which you are supposed to be).

It also bears mentioning that adverse counsel may direct you to respond to certain questions with a simple "yes" or "no" answer. However, if you are unable to respond in that fashion, you can not be forced to do so, despite such instruction.

Jurors in the courtroom, like people you encounter every day in the real world, admire candor. Evasiveness is not a quality to which individuals favorably respond. If you attempt to answer questions in a direct fashion and do so repeatedly, you will gain the jury's respect. This is a most important step in achieving the type of rapport with jurors that will place you in a position to convince them of the merit of your opinions as you try to withstand cross-examination.

More important, to the extent that juries equate candor with honesty, the significance of question responsiveness cannot be underestimated. An evasive witness (or at least one who appears evasive) will be squarely rejected by the jury. Should that occur, notwithstanding the relative strength of the expert's opinions, the likelihood that the jury will embrace that expert's views is remote. If the expert impresses the jury as honest, the battle to gain juror acceptance is likely won.

Thus, the cumulative effect of multiple non-responsive answers to examination can be devastating. Since the liability expert is typically the lynchpin of the defendant's case, rejection of the expert by the jury for such conduct will likely destroy any chance of trial success. Remember, if a subject is sufficiently significant, the retaining attorney will always have an opportunity on redirect examination to go back to those matters addressed by adverse counsel in an effort to have you more fully explain testimony deliberately restricted by cross-examination. Do not risk damage to yourself by trying to circumvent the limitations intentionally imposed by cross-examination. Such effort will create more problems than it will solve.

Interpersonal Connection

People are people. This most elemental of axioms has real application to the courtroom. As an expert, it is your job to convince a group of strangers that you are worthy of belief. Achieving this goal requires that the expert "connect" with each member of the jury on an interpersonal level. Outside the courtroom, this task is far easier to achieve. In fact, the "connection" of which I speak occurs with some frequency. It occurs regularly in your personal life, and of course, it happens routinely in your professional life.

In a typical practice, the opportunity to connect with people exists every day and often. Each time you see a patient, you "connect". This human interaction is unforced, natural and typically successful. If you were not capable of connecting with patients, new and old, you would not survive professionally. It's really no different in the courtroom. In fact, speak to the jury as you would to patients.

Whatever it is you do to establish and maintain relationships in your profession is what you must try to accomplish in court, albeit in an accelerated manner. That effort is defined by perhaps the most basic of human interaction— conversation. Think about what you do during conversation to communicate your thoughts, to convince, to persuade. Those are the things you must be willing to do as a trial witness.

Unlike encounters in the real world, however, those that occur in court are the result of a deliberate design. The environment is created by circumstance to achieve the resolution of disputes. The participants, somewhat involuntarily, converge to air issues and to foster "debate" so as to permit previously unidentified individuals (jurors) to "arbitrate" disagreements and fashion remedies. It is in this environment that you are summoned to aid in the resolution process and to that end you must effectively "communicate". Unlike the more natural and familiar forums in which you daily encounter people, courtroom communication is only permitted in accordance with certain "rules" of conduct and you as a trial witness must function within those "rules". Persuasive "conversation", therefore, is more difficult. Within the confines of this environment, however, human connections can nevertheless be forged.

Perhaps the most effective method is to address each juror as an individual. That is, rather than to generally look at the jury as a group, a deliberate effort must be made to develop a one-on-one "dialog" with each juror. The goal is to make each jury member feel as though you are speaking directly to him or her. The expert can accomplish this by looking at each juror for a few moments while testifying as though he or she is being individually addressed. Given the typical length of direct examination, this likely can be done repeatedly during direct testimony. The juror to whom the expert is speaking will feel engaged by the testimony and consequently will respond favorably to the expert.

Of course, the "yes" or "no" responses typically sought of experts by adverse counsel during cross-examination will limit opportunities to speak to the jury at length. However, when they do occur, the expert should answer such questions of the opposing attorney by talking directly to the jury.

A second and related aspect of the interpersonal encounter is eye contact. While speaking directly to each juror, it is imperative that the expert make eye contact. Again, direct testimony will consume a significant amount of time—certainly enough time for the expert to look into the eyes of each juror on multiple occasions. The expert must make a conscious effort in this regard. If the expert is able to make and sustain eye contact, the jurors will probably feel more comfortable with him or her. If the witness looks away from the individual jurors, it is unlikely that the expert will make the necessary connection.

Be careful to avoid appearing as though your head is on a swivel. If your response to a question posed during direct examination allows for but a brief response, there is no need to turn to the jury before answering. To do so and to do so frequently will make your testimony look contrived and can only serve to damage an otherwise credible presentation.

Testimony Content

The content of an expert's responses to courtroom examination must be understandable, if not simple. Remember, the individuals you are addressing are not professional colleagues. Jurors will typically have no educational or practical foundation upon which to draw in an effort to understand what will customarily be rather complicated and complex concepts. At best, a juror's knowledge base usually will be limited to that gained from being a patient. Consequently, the expert must avoid defining difficult precepts with equally difficult explanations. The process requires "plain talking".

If you have taught or currently teach students or residents, you likely understand the "plain talking" notion, which is even more important in the context of trial testimony. Although you may consider the courtroom a classroom for the limited purpose of conveying your thoughts during a single "lecture", the challenge presented in the courtroom is somewhat different from that offered in the classroom.

Unlike those taught in the classroom, the "students" in the courtroom are not there by choice. By and large, they have no science background. They are not seeking a career in the very field you have selected as your own. In sum, they will not recognize or quickly absorb principles with which you routinely deal and they are not provided with textbooks to review before, during and after your presentation so as to permit concept reinforcement.

As a result, you must be able to convey your thoughts in a manner that optimizes the relatively brief time you have with the jury. Not only must the jurors understand what you are saying, they must recall your testimony, or at least the most salient portions of it, when they deliberate, which in most trials will be days after you have testified. The more difficult the subject matter, the greater the challenge. It is not enough that you have the credentials and experience to know about the discrete issues presented by the case. Without "talking down" to the jurors, you must also be able to explain those issues so that the jury understands and remembers. To that end, use universally recognizable terms. Where necessary, definitions of concepts must be provided. In sum, deliberate care must be taken to render otherwise mysterious matters obvious and clear.

An expert may unwittingly respond to questions about complex concepts with vague, meandering and/or unduly lengthy responses. Frankly, a jury's tolerance for expert testimony provided in this fashion is limited—no, very limited. Certainly, this can happen even to the most experienced of expert witnesses. However, if you are speaking directly to the jury, as you must and in the manner already described, you should be able to recognize when you have "lost" your audience. If the jurors' eyes appear to glaze over, the need to speak plainly becomes acute. In the alternative, if you notice the occasional approving head nods, you likely are effectively peppering your testimony with sufficient explanations and definitions. From the jury's perspective, simple testimony about complex matters is easier to understand and ultimately, easier to recall.

Trial Aids

Bringing your testimony to life is a key to persuading the jury. Given the proposition that, by definition, the content of expert testimony is beyond the knowledge of the average juror, enhancing that testimony indeed is a trial objective.

Accomplishing that goal should be the focus of discussions with retaining counsel well in advance of your trial appearance. In my opinion, trial aids are a means to that end and fall into two categories—verbal aids and physical aids.

Verbal aids are easily incorporated into trial testimony and at times are spontaneous. They typically take the form of analogies to life experiences that are easily identifiable by jurors. For example, if the subject matter is orthopedic surgery, the expert may liken bones, orthopedic hardware and surgical instruments to wood, screws and shop tools. Certainly, I have more easily understood the surgical procedures discussed by experts in those terms and often have noticed outward physical manifestations of juror understanding (such as greater attentiveness and head nodding) when such analogies are used. Other examples are likening tendons to rubber bands and equating the impeded blood flow in an obstructed blood vessel to the water flow in a kinked garden hose. Some analogies are quite simple and some are less so. Some may be devised prior to the expert's court appearance and deliberately injected into the expert's testimony at the appropriate time and some may come to mind during testimony. Either way, analogies drawn from common experience invariably assist in the jury's understanding of the expert's testimony at the time offered and are easily recalled at the later and critical time of jury deliberations.

Make certain, however, that the verbal analogies you employ are those that can be offered in gender-mixed company. No matter how "cute" or "catchy", avoid those that can be interpreted as sexist or gender-biased.

As an example, in an effort to explain a medical condition, my seasoned expert spontaneously and surprisingly indicated that his description of the condition's severity could be easily understood by using a scale of "1 to 10", 10 being at the ultimate end of the range, "like Bo Derek". Those of you who understand the reference should also recognize that this sexist remark was ill-advised. I internally cringed at the moment, acutely sensitive to the expert's comment. My hope, however, was that the gender-mixed jury would ignore and ultimately forget it.

The second type of trial aid is the physical one and can include anatomical models, drawings, photos, videos, blow-ups, displays, PowerPoint slides and computer-generated images. If there is one thing about which I am certain, it is the value of such demonstrative evidence. It serves to teach a juror in a manner that no spoken word alone can accomplish. Physical trial aids complement the verbal presentation and increase the jury's interest. They should be a planned focal point of the expert's direct testimony, which will bring to life what might otherwise be perceived as boring, dry, uninter-esting or overwhelmingly complex. Once used during your direct testimony, these aids will be available to you for use during cross-examination as circumstances warrant. In fact, you may gain control of the cross-examination by offering to use such exhibits during your responses.

In sum, demonstrative evidence makes you and your court-room presentation better. It stands to reason, therefore, that you should consider the use of physical trial aids in connec-tion with your testimony whenever and wherever possible.

Every courtroom is (or at least should be) equipped with a large pad on an easel. At a minimum, you should use it to make anatomical drawings to help explain your testimony. Of course, if you are incapable of effectively drawing parts of the anatomy (and many highly regarded and exceptionally competent practitioners simply cannot draw) don't attempt this in court before a jury. Instead, use an illustration that you already have in your office for patient education or can locate in textbooks, journal articles or even on a website. (I am par-ticularly partial to the Frank Netter, M.D. published collection of anatomical illustrations, which are beautifully detailed, in color and labeled.)

Three-dimensional models of the anatomy are also a favor-ite of mine and typically are fascinating to jurors. If you have a relevant anatomical model in your office, recommend to retaining counsel that it be used during the course of your testimony. Because of its three-dimensional value, a model is probably one of the most effective aids at trial.

Enlarging treatment records into poster size exhibits or creating PowerPoint slides may also prove helpful. Expert testimony about matters recorded in a hospital or office chart will be lifeless and dull. However, placing an enlargement of those notes before the jury during expert testimony will undoubtedly increase juror interest in their content and will render otherwise mundane expert review of such entries more appealing.

With the proliferation of sophisticated computer-based software, attention should be paid to their use by experts at trial. Laptops can be brought to court and with the aid of a projector and a large monitor (typically found in courtrooms) or portable screen, PowerPoint presentations and computer-generated images can be used during expert testimony in much the same way as more conventional drawings, pictures and models are used. Once again, the goal is to render the expert's testimony more understandable and interesting. To the extent that the computer can assist in that process, it too should be considered as a valuable trial aid.

Litigation support firms, medical illustrators, pharmaceutical companies, reproduction or graphics shops, photography studios or photocopy stores can provide many if not all of the trial aids discussed and can be contacted by retaining counsel after you have discussed and selected the appropriate exhibits.

In addition, many manufacturers of medical devices, instruments and prosthetic components produce and distribute videos of their products and their use. Although typically created for review by practitioners who may be influenced to purchase and/or use such products, videos of this type, without the audio component, may serve a useful trial purpose. If the matter involves, for example, a certain prosthetic implant

and the manufacturer of that item has produced an informa-
tional video for practitioners to show to patients, it may prove
educational at trial and may serve to enhance the expert's
testimony. Assuming there are no evidential impediments to its
use, this aid will likely be beneficial at trial.

Intangibles

In addition to the very palpable qualities already discussed,
there exists one final value worthy of note. Although mentioned last, its location in this chapter is not intended to
minimize its importance.

As is the case in everyday life, positive human response
to experiencing a new event or meeting a new individual is
dependent upon favorable stimulation of the senses. That is to
say, often the "good feeling" enjoyed, results not so much from
an intellectual reaction but rather from a quasi-emotional one.
If you feel "comfortable" speaking to a new acquaintance, that
individual by word and/or by deed has triggered a positive
response on many levels. As an expert, it is imperative that
you secure a similar reaction in the jurors you seek to impress.

In the process of accomplishing or at least attempting to
accomplish the goals recited above, the expert must portray
himself as an authority on the subject at hand without appearing as an advocate for the defendant. The expert must always
be a neutral, objective, third-party examiner of the facts.
The expert must be somewhat detached from the matter and
not seem to be championing the cause of the defendant on
whose behalf the expert has been retained. That of course is
the job of the defense attorney. The expert's alignment with
that party must appear to be borne of a dispassionate assessment of the events rather than a financially motivated acqui-
escence in an attorney's request for assistance. In this way, the
expert will likely evoke a "comfortable" reaction by the jury.
That is, the jurors will tend to accept the notion that the witness

really is an "expert", one whose opinions are prompted by a true understanding of the issues and whose presence is not the result of some "agenda", be it political, economic or otherwise.

Of course, the expert must really believe in the opinions advanced in court or at least sound like it. Just like laughter, compelling comments fervently offered by an expert in court can be contagious. If you testify with conviction, it is likely that the jury or certain of its members will find themselves recalling, and more important, reiterating your statements in the jury room during deliberations, when it really counts. Indeed, transforming once uninformed jurors into opinion-spouting disciples is the goal. Always remember that you must engage them during your testimony. Put the jurors at ease and then draw them in.

Chapter 4

Case Participation

With some exception, malpractice cases require the expert's participation in certain anticipated and defined ways. The role of the expert is dictated by the jurisdiction in which the matter is venued, and although there will be some variation from state to state, you can expect a fairly uniform experience no matter where the lawsuit is filed.

Telephone Conferences

The defense expert's initial contact with a case typically occurs as a result of a telephone call from the attorney representing a defendant, in an already existing suit. Frequently, a plaintiff's attorney must obtain an affidavit signed by an individual who practices in the defendant's specialty and who is familiar with the applicable standard of care indicating that a review of records reveals that the named defendant committed malpractice. This Affidavit of Merit, as it's called in New Jersey, is prepared by the plaintiff's lawyer and contains the language required by law. Without it, the court will dismiss the matter. As a result, a plaintiff's attorney will typically retain a liability expert before a suit is instituted. Defense counsel may not need the services of a liability expert until the case is underway.

During that first telephone conversation, the defense lawyer will generally outline the facts, reveal the names of the parties, identify the venue of the suit and indicate the intended purpose in retaining you. Understand that successful prosecution of a malpractice action by a plaintiff requires that liability, causation and damages be established. Generally speaking, a plaintiff must prove liability, i.e., that a practitioner deviated from the accepted standard of care and causation, i.e., that the alleged deviation caused injury. Finally, a plaintiff must establish damages, i.e., the nature and extent of the injury caused by the malpractice. Your role might be to offer defense opinions about the issues of liability, causation or damages or some combination of these components. Consequently, time should be devoted to discussing the issues you are comfortable addressing, given your practice area.

In some venues, a defense attorney may retain you for the sole purpose of preparing a "pocket report" critical of a co-defendant practitioner. This occurs when it is anticipated that an expert may be needed to testify at trial about that co-defendant's departures from the standard of care. If that co-defendant settles in advance of trial, the testimony of the "pocket expert" can be introduced and considered by the jury. If both the defendant and the settling co-defendant are determined to be culpable, the adverse verdict against the defendant could be reduced by the percentage of responsibility attributed by the jury to the settling co-defendant. Of course, no additional money can be obtained from the settling co-defendant because the plaintiff's claims against the co-defendant were previously settled.

If you have an interest in participating, your fee structure should be discussed, and assuming that the attorney retains your services, documents thereafter will be supplied to you for review. Before agreeing to take the case, you should inquire as to the date by which you must complete your review of the materials. If counsel needs an expeditious assessment, you must know this up front.

Document Review

The stage of the litigation will dictate the documents you will be forwarded for assessment. If the matter is in its infancy, it is likely that you will only receive a copy of the Complaint and copies of the treatment records (possibly including imaging studies of various types) concerning the care under scrutiny and treatment after the alleged malpractice. If the lawsuit has been pending for some time, in addition to these basic documents, you probably will receive copies of additional "discovery" material. Discovery documents commonly include copies of the various parties' written answers to interrogatories (questions), deposition transcripts and miscellaneous documents in the possession of the parties' attorneys. In jurisdictions where service of expert reports is required, you will receive a copy of a report or reports generated by the plaintiff's expert(s).

Some attorneys consider it appropriate to transmit materials with a summary or outline of the relevant facts to facilitate the expert's review. Many don't. I firmly believe that written summaries are unnecessary and I do not recommend that you request one. To the extent that you require a summary of the relevant events, ask for it verbally when the attorney first calls you. Remember that your analysis of the case must be based on the untainted facts revealed by a review of the treatment records, interrogatory answers, deposition transcripts and the documents exchanged by counsel. If you rely to any extent upon lawyer-generated chronologies in the formation of your opinions, your conclusions may be suspect. In some venues, such written summaries contained in the expert's file may be properly requested by adverse counsel at an expert's deposition and/or during the expert's trial testimony. If the facts are even slightly skewed to favor the defendant on whose behalf you are conducting your review, the adverse attorney will discover the tainted summary and reveal it as such to the jury through cross-examination. As a result, the independence of your assessment will be questioned.

It also is recommended that you not make notes directly on the documents supplied unless absolutely necessary. Notes on the materials are a potentially fertile topic of examination. For this reason, avoid making written comments that are or can be interpreted as adverse to the defendant on whose behalf you have been retained.

Notes on separate sheets of paper are also discouraged for the same reason. If you refer to such notes during deposition or trial, adverse counsel is entitled to see them. If your notes are but a simple recitation of certain facts, an inspection by adverse counsel will be uneventful. If the notes contain remarks that can be construed as damaging to the defendant on whose behalf you have been retained, scrutiny by opposing counsel may prove problematic. Of course, I recognize that factually complex cases or those generating voluminous documents may require you to prepare written notes emphasizing or highlighting portions of the material reviewed. To the extent you may be obligated to produce these writings, it is recommended that you create such sheets sparingly and never make a note adverse to the interests of the defendant on whose behalf you have been retained.

However, if the notes serve as a prelude to report preparation and can be construed as a draft of that report, they may not have to be produced, no matter their content. Commonly, drafts which precede the final product are not discoverable and notes which are generated as part of the "collaborative process" with counsel may be equally protected from disclosure.

Nevertheless, depending upon the jurisdiction in which the case is venued, perhaps the best solution to the note-taking conundrum prior to actual report preparation is the computer.

If you make notes in a computer file, you can use those entries to serve as a rough outline of your thoughts that ultimately can be merged into a report, leaving nothing behind for adverse counsel to review.

Case Assessment

Following your assessment of the file, you should telephone defense counsel with the results of that review. Assuming your opinions allow you to serve as an expert on behalf of that attorney's client, this telephone exchange is vital. The conversation should focus on the issues, your understanding of the facts and the opinions you have formulated based on those facts. Of course, if your opinions are of little or no assistance to retaining counsel, your service will likely end at this point. If, however, your assessment favors the defendant on whose behalf you have reviewed the case, your next task likely may be to prepare a report.

Assuming a defensible review, a written report will be requested by defense counsel in jurisdictions like New Jersey and upon receipt will be forwarded to opposing counsel. In states like New York, a formal report will rarely be requested as there is no procedural requirement that a party serve an expert report on the adverse litigant in advance of trial. In fact, expert reports are discouraged by attorneys in some jurisdictions who fear that they may be discoverable by adverse counsel in certain limited circumstances. When required, however, the report should recite the salient facts, the expert's opinions and the relationship between both.

In states where the expert report must be served on all other attorneys involved in the litigation, expect that the adverse experts will read it. The importance of the expert report has already been discussed and the specific contents of the expert report will be addressed in later sections. For now, it is enough to understand that participation as an expert may require a written expression of your thoughts prepared in letter format.

Literature Review

Literature in a malpractice case serves a variety of purposes. At a minimum, it can and should be used to educate defense counsel about the practice area and the specific topics involved. Literature can be used to reeducate a malpractice defendant about obscure but litigation-related issues. Perhaps most important, literature dramatically enhances a litigant's position in a malpractice trial. Of this, I am certain.

Consequently, if relevant published material exists, it is imperative that it is located. Oftentimes, experts are aware of journal articles or textbook references that are both relevant and/or supportive. (Better yet, the expert may have authored a pertinent work.) If so, the expert should identify and/or provide copies of the material. In other instances, a retaining attorney may ask an expert to either conduct a literature search or assist counsel in obtaining copies of certain pieces of literature.

To the extent timely literature does exist and is entirely helpful to the defense of a matter, it should be used by the expert to bolster opinions offered. Of course, if you are aware of literature that contradicts the position advanced by the defendant or if a search reveals such material, it must be brought to the attention of retaining counsel. As well, if you have published literature that runs counter to the defendant's position in a given case, you must alert the retaining attorney.

Supplemental Document Review

After providing your opinions to retaining counsel, whether or not in written report form, the ongoing litigation will thereafter generate additional documents that will require your review. For example, updated treatment records of those still providing care to the plaintiff will continue to be gathered and reports prepared by practitioners retained to conduct IMEs (Independent Medical Examinations) of various types may be obtained.

Such materials are properly supplied to the expert for assessment and analysis, typically prompting additional opinions and the need for preparation of a supplemental report in states where written reports are a necessity. To the extent such additional documents do not significantly affect your previously expressed opinions, nothing more than a brief letter identifying the new materials and so stating will suffice. If the supplemental documents require a detailed analysis, the form of your addendum report may track your original one. In either instance, the retaining lawyer will provide some guidance as to how best to proceed.

Deposition Testimony

After the attorneys have exchanged the reports of their experts, as frequently occurs, depositions of the experts are conducted. Customarily (although not necessarily required by local court rules), the plaintiff's expert is deposed first and the defense expert some time later.

Depositions occur outside the courtroom but can prove as important as in-court proceedings. Although the details of the deposition will be discussed later, I want to address certain aspects of the deposition here.

Expert depositions historically have been conducted in the retaining attorney's office or in the expert's office. During COVID-19, however, almost all depositions have occurred remotely. Some jurisdictions do not require the exchange of expert reports and consequently, depositions of experts are never conducted. Many states allow for expert depositions and attorneys usually use this discovery tool.

The deposition is a verbal question and answer session attended by the expert, lawyers for the parties and a court reporter (and infrequently the litigants themselves as observers). Questions based upon the expert's credentials, the nature of the expert's practice and the contents of the expert's report are verbally posed by adverse counsel and occasionally by the attorneys of other defendants. The expert answers orally under oath and everything said at the deposition is recorded by a court reporter retained by the attorney conducting the deposition and thereafter prepared in transcript form.

In the typical case, months pass between the preparation of an expert report and the deposition of the expert. Accordingly, it is essential that the expert review the file materials before appearing for deposition. It also is recommended that a pre-deposition conference with retaining counsel be conducted to discuss key issues, review relevant records and analyze the details of the expert's opinions.

General Assistance

Once retained, the expert likely will be needed to serve in a variety of ways beyond those mentioned above. Throughout the course of the case, litigation-driven events will require the expert's input. Where expert reports are exchanged, an expert is commonly consulted with respect to the opinions expressed in the adverse expert's report.

If the matter in which you are participating is venued in a state that permits expert depositions, you may be enlisted to aid defense counsel in preparation of the plaintiff's expert's deposition. This may require review of written materials and conferences with retaining counsel.

Trial Stage

All roads lead to the trial. Typically, it is the culmination of years of effort. It also is the ultimate forum for presenting the expert's opinions. Trial details will be discussed later.

For now, it is enough that you appreciate that unless the Complaint is dismissed (by the plaintiff voluntarily or by the court involuntarily) or the case is settled, the matter will be tried. Consequently, when you embark on your expert career, you should understand that you likely will become a trial witness. As I have mentioned, this responsibility usually will require you to take time away from your practice to appear in court at a time and place that might not be convenient. It also will require you to again become familiar enough with the details of the case to comfortably discuss them in court before a jury.

In lieu of live courtroom testimony, there are occasions when video-recorded testimony of an expert is presented to the jury by counsel. Although a live appearance is almost always more effective, scheduling snafus may create the need to record an expert. Such testimony usually is recorded at the retaining attorney's office but can be scheduled in the expert's office. Video-recorded testimony mimics a live presentation. All that is missing are the judge and jury. Nevertheless, it requires the same pre-appearance preparation.

Chapter 5

The Expert Opinion

Critical to the prosecution or defense of almost every malpractice case is the liability expert opinion. Without it, a plaintiff will be unable to pursue or at least sustain a malpractice action and a defendant will be unable to defend one. There are occasions, although few, when an expert opinion is unnecessary. For example, under the doctrine of *res ipsa loquitur,* which means literally "the thing speaks for itself", a jury may reasonably conclude that an alleged injury would not have occurred absent the defendant's misconduct. This doctrine rarely applies in malpractice matters because the expert opinion is almost always needed to address the propriety of what occurred.

Another exception to the liability expert opinion requirement exists where the "common knowledge" doctrine applies. Here, the law recognizes that there may be situations where lay individuals based on their everyday experience can determine if there has been a departure from the accepted standard of care. Application of this doctrine requires professional conduct so clearly wanting that it is obvious to a layperson.

By way of example, if right ear surgery is scheduled for a pediatric patient for mastoiditis and surgery is performed by a pediatric otolaryngologist, a less than optimal result may prompt the filing of a malpractice suit. If the surgery was neither ill-conceived nor improperly performed, there will be no basis for a malpractice action, unless, of course, the surgery was performed on the left ear instead of the right. Such was a case that I defended. As you might imagine, the plaintiffs did not retain an expert to address the issue of negligence. It was conceded that the problem ear was the right ear and not the left one. By surgically treating the wrong ear, the defendant practitioner clearly had deviated from the standard of care. The jury did not need, and the law did not require, the assistance of expert testimony to so find.

You would think that a case like this would be settled, rather than tried. After all, my client and I both understood that a trial would result in an adverse verdict. By eliminating the need to retain the services of a liability expert, the plaintiffs (parents of the patient) through their attorney would be able to pursue the matter inexpensively, dispense with the need for a lengthy trial and secure a monetary settlement. The plaintiffs and/or their attorney, however, demanded an excessive sum of money to resolve the matter. Interestingly, it was conceded that the surgery did not cause any real injury to the ear that was the subject of surgery and probably improved its condition. In fact, according to the defendant, the surgical ear also had a problem that likely would have required surgery in the near future. Our defense, therefore, was that damages were limited. Unable to convince the plaintiffs' lawyer that he and his clients were significantly overvaluing the case, I realized that the matter would have to be tried. Although my client and I understood that a "no cause" verdict was impossible, I also believed that the likelihood of a jury verdict in excess of the settlement demand was slim. Indeed, the jury returned a verdict for the plaintiffs, but the monetary award was half of the settlement demand.

Verbal Opinion

As mentioned, retention of a liability expert commonly begins with a telephone call to a practitioner placed by defense counsel, who will recite the facts and allegations and then inquire as to whether the practitioner has an interest in reviewing the case. With an affirmative response from the expert, the defense attorney will then ask: "Did the defendant depart from the applicable standard of care and cause injury?" Based on the telephone call, the expert may be able to express a liability opinion—or may not. Often, a preliminary oral response to this question is possible with the caveat that a review of relevant records may prompt a different reply. Even without a firm substantive response, an expression of support for the defendant practitioner will usually result in retention of the expert for the purpose of reviewing the written materials and formulating a liability opinion.

An expert may be retained to address the issues of causation or damages rather than liability. If the issue of concern is causation, the pivotal question asked of a potential expert may be: "Did the defendant's conduct cause damage to the patient?" If the damage claim is the focus, the lawyer may ask: "Can you identify, characterize or quantify the patient's injuries?" Again, without having scrutinized the relevant records, the expert may offer only a preliminary opinion. If it is encouraging, counsel likely will retain the expert and forward the appropriate documents for review.

Of course, as the litigation develops and additional materials are supplied, the need for verbal input will be ongoing.

Written Report

Typically, the liability expert report is critical and is written in the form of a letter to retaining counsel on professional letterhead. To the extent that it embodies opinions crucial to the litigation, its importance cannot be underestimated. Although the report will reflect the individual writing style of its author, reports should all contain certain information organized in a recognizable format. In my practice, I have seen thousands of liability expert reports, some better than others. It is up to you to create a report that effectively delivers your thoughts. Given the subject matter usually addressed, the report will necessarily contain highly technical concepts and terms. The key, however, is to craft the report so that the reader will understand your opinions and the basis for them. Without question, the more experience you gain preparing expert reports, the better you will be as a draftsman.

The stage of the litigation will dictate the general report type. An initial defense liability report customarily will be the most encompassing of all reports. It will embody the expert's analysis of the key documents and likely will contain opinions crucial to the defense. Reports thereafter prepared by the same expert are usually supplemental and less comprehensive. They typically do not review the facts (already recited in the initial report) and normally are confined to an assessment of additional documents obtained by the retaining attorney during pretrial discovery or an analysis of additional issues raised by those documents or statements made by parties or witnesses at deposition. Consequently, the format of such supplemental reports will be governed by their purpose. They usually are shorter than the initial report, and although their preparation may benefit from reliance on the format discussed below, addendum reports need not strictly comply with such outline. In fact, at times, the supplemental liability report may simply identify the additional documents reviewed and contain a statement that they "do not alter my opinions as previously expressed".

The length of the initial liability report and each of its sections will be dictated by the nature of the case. If the matter is factually complex and/or encompasses complicated treatment issues, it is reasonable to expect that the report will be longer rather than shorter. As a general proposition, I have rarely seen a comprehensive initial expert report much less than two single-spaced typewritten letter-size pages. Even the simplest of matters likely will necessitate such a report.

Although headings need not be used in the report, at a minimum, there are certain recognizable components of a properly prepared initial expert report:

- Materials reviewed
- Facts
- Issues
- Opinions
- Foundation for opinions
- Ultimate conclusion

Let's analyze each.

Materials Reviewed

The report should initially acknowledge receipt of the materials supplied by identifying them. Although some experts (experienced and inexperienced alike) may recite only a partial list or state that "various documents have been furnished for review", it is preferable that each item be listed. If the documents reviewed were supplied by counsel at various points in time (and even if they weren't), a report listing in one place all materials furnished will be of help if and when that expert is deposed and is asked to identify the documents reviewed in the formulation of opinions as contained in the initial report. It will be of immense benefit also at trial, when a similar question is posed. If you don't know or cannot easily and quickly provide the answer, it will suggest that you are not thorough and in command of the materials. Although the expert can always refer back to retaining counsel's transmittal letters, testimony regarding this subject then becomes disjointed. Avoid this simply by itemizing the documents in the report.

Facts

The next section should recite the salient facts. Although the facts may be gleaned from multiple records and documents, with occasional exception, it is not necessary to identify in the report the source of each fact. A chronological narrative based upon an understanding of the facts as revealed by the various materials is best. Although some experts provide a summary of the facts as contained in each key document, this is not the preferred approach. Nor is it recommended that the report's length be extended by including superfluous facts irrelevant to the issues in dispute.

Issues

The very reason you have been retained is to address the issues raised by the litigation. If you are a liability expert, it is expected that you will here identify the claims that stem from the treatment provided by the defendant practitioner. Alleged acts of commission and omission should be noted. At times, a plaintiff will advance a lack of informed consent claim asserting that the defendant failed to completely disclose the material risks of or the reasonable alternatives to the subject treatment. Generally speaking, a jury will decide whether material risks or viable treatment options were withheld and, if so, whether the reasonably prudent patient in the plaintiff's position would have consented to the treatment if disclosure was complete. Consequently, where an informed consent issue exists, the expert must identify it. The degree to which the defense expert must discuss the informed consent claim is dependant on the jurisdiction's legal requirements and is variable. Guidance from defense counsel as to this issue will be needed.

As with the other portions of the report, this section is best written in paragraph form. An outline or listing format may be appropriate in certain situations but should be the exception, rather than the rule, in report drafting.

Typically, by the time a defense expert report is needed, the specific deviations allegedly attributable to the defendant have already been identified in the plaintiff's liability expert report. As a liability expert, you must address each and every deviation cited by the plaintiff's expert. Omitting an issue can prove disastrous as it may preclude you from offering opinion testimony about that point at trial.

If you have been retained exclusively as a causation or damages expert, these guidelines are equally applicable. Although the issues in such circumstance are different, your general approach to report construction should not be. In this report section, you should always address each and every issue.

Opinions

Here is where you should fully offer your opinions about all the issues. Completely analyze the disputed topics and offer your conclusions as to each issue. In doing so, however, resist the temptation to write too much. Say just enough to adequately explain yourself without becoming repetitive, meandering or confusing. Be concise. Simply make your point and move on. Recognize that you are writing a report for defense counsel to understand, not a journal article for professional review. Know too that attorneys appreciate brevity. With all that we have to read, digest and recall in the representation of a litigant, a retained expert who can write concisely is welcome.

Foundation for Opinions

An expert's opinions are no stronger than the foundation upon which they are based. If the foundation is tenuous, the opinions will falter. The report must relate the expert's thinking to the facts found in the materials supplied for review. It is not enough that the expert's conceptual reasoning is flawless. For the opinion to pass muster, it must be built upon facts of record.

By way of example, if a lawsuit advanced by a plaintiff against a surgeon includes a claim for failure to respond to a postoperative patient rapidly deteriorating during the overnight hours, a plaintiff's expert will likely offer an opinion that the surgeon had an obligation consistent with the standard of care to act affirmatively. That expert would likely identify tests that should have been ordered, medications that should have been administered and consultations that should have been requested. In the face of the defendant surgeon's failure to do anything, the expert will probably offer a scathing assessment of the defendant's conduct and be reasonably convincing in doing so—unless the expert failed to note that the hospital chart lacked any indication that the surgeon was ever contacted about the patient's deteriorating status. Although the expert's recitation of the standard of care and analysis of the surgeon's departure from that standard might be theoretically unassailable, the absence of a necessary factual predicate—the surgeon's knowledge—will be the expert's undoing.

Conversely, if that same expert had been retained on behalf of the defendant surgeon and he offered the opinion that the practitioner complied with the standard of care based on the assumed fact that his inaction resulted from the lack of information supplied to him by the hospital nurses in attendance, he better not miss the entry in the Nurses' Notes that recites otherwise. Again, the expert's defense of the surgeon may be conceptually compelling, but if it is not built upon a factual foundation, it will crumble.

Ultimate Conclusion

This section of the report is typically no longer than a paragraph or two and may even be as short as two or three sentences. A plaintiff's expert's conclusion of this type will often read as follows: "Based on the above, it is my opinion that the defendant deviated from the accepted standard of care in the treatment of the plaintiff and that as a direct result, the plaintiff was injured. It further is my opinion that the plaintiff's injuries as described are permanent in nature. I offer these opinions within a reasonable degree of medical probability."

In some jurisdictions, the deviation opinion should incorporate the term "certainty" rather than "probability". The retaining attorney will guide you as to the applicable requirement.

Yours, however, will typically resemble the following: "Based on the above, it is my opinion that the defendant did not deviate from the accepted standard of care at any time during treatment of the plaintiff and that nothing the defendant did caused injury to the plaintiff. It further is my opinion that the plaintiff's present condition as described above is the result of events in which the defendant played no part. I offer these opinions within a reasonable degree of medical probability."

Again, "certainty" may be the operative term, depending upon the jurisdiction's requirements.

Independent Medical Examination

Oftentimes, a key issue in a malpractice matter apart from the alleged malpractice is the plaintiff's physical condition. This issue may arise in the context of examining causation and/or damages. In the former circumstance, the jury must determine whether the condition of the plaintiff is the result of the criticized conduct of the defendant. In the latter situation, the jury must evaluate the full nature and extent of the injury of which the plaintiff complains. Frequently, both causation and damages are affected by evidence about a plaintiff's current condition. Consequently, experts on both sides typically are retained to conduct an IME (Independent

Medical Examination) of the plaintiff. On occasion, a treating practitioner will be retained by the plaintiff to serve as the liability expert. Since the practitioner is already familiar with the plaintiff's condition, in that instance, liability as well as causation and/or damages issues can be easily addressed by a single expert. This occurs rarely, however, because a liability expert who has an ongoing relationship with the plaintiff may not appear objective.

Although not always the case, at times, the independent examining physician may also serve as the liability expert. The facts of a given case will dictate to defense counsel whether it is advisable for one person to serve as an expert on liability and damages, or liability and causation, or liability, damages and causation.

By way of example, if the defendant is a pediatrician who allegedly failed to timely diagnose hip dysplasia in a newborn resulting in multiple surgeries when the patient became a toddler, an IME to address the damages issue may benefit the defendant. Since the malpractice claim involves the conduct of a pediatrician, the liability experts retained by the parties should be pediatricians, not orthopedists. However, the IME should be performed by a pediatric orthopedist because the consequences of the alleged malpractice would be within such a practitioner's area of expertise.

Similarly, if the malpractice claim concerns a neurologic injury to the brachial plexus following an obstetrician's inability to deliver a newborn due to a condition where the anterior shoulder cannot pass below the pubic bone, known as shoulder dystocia, the liability expert should be an obstetrician. However, since the resulting injury is some degree of paralysis of the arm, forearm and/or hand, that is, Erb's and/or Klumpke's Palsy, the IME to assess damages should be performed by a pediatric neurologist.

In each of these examples, the participation of practitioners in two different disciplines is required. In each instance, the liability expert cannot conduct the IME and the physician conducting the IME cannot offer opinions about deviation from or compliance with the applicable standard of care.

A different situation may arise in an action alleging a negligently performed hip replacement by an orthopedic surgeon. There, the need for an orthopedic expert to discuss the standard of care and alleged departures from that standard is obvious. If permanency is an issue (and it always is in such a matter), an IME will likely be necessary. Inasmuch as the current condition of the plaintiff will be orthopedic in nature, the IME should also be performed by an orthopedic surgeon. Since the liability question is properly handled by an orthopedic surgeon, it makes sense that the liability expert also conduct the IME. Consequently, only a single expert is needed and the report prepared by that expert should address all the issues—liability (deviation from the standard of care), causation (the connection between the alleged deviation and the resultant injury or condition) and damages (the nature, extent and duration of the injury or condition).

The possibility exists, therefore, that you may serve as the liability expert in a given case, and another practitioner specializing in a different field may perform the IME and act as the causation and/or damages expert. It is equally possible that you might serve as the liability, causation and damages expert. The particular facts and allegations in a given matter will direct whether multiple experts are needed.

Potential Pitfalls

It is impossible to discuss all the potential problems that might arise during the review of materials or while generating a report. Certain difficulties will be peculiar to a given case. If you follow the guidelines above, however, problems you might otherwise encounter will be minimized. Still, there are certain problems that can occur and that are worth mentioning.

Issue Identification

Crucial to a solid and complete expert opinion is identification of all issues involved in the litigation. It is absolutely essential that you isolate the acts of alleged malpractice attributable to the defendant on whose behalf you have been retained, including the previously mentioned and typically troublesome lack of informed consent claim, if applicable, and discuss each with clarity. If a plaintiff's expert fails to uncover all of the defendant's conduct that might be criticized, that expert may weaken the plaintiff's case and dilute its economic value. Similarly, as a defense expert, if you neglect to fully evaluate the entirety of the defendant's conduct, you may compromise his or her defense. In jurisdictions where expert reports are served by counsel on the adverse party, the defense expert's job is simplified. He need only review the plaintiff's expert report to ascertain which aspects of the practitioner's care are at issue and respond accordingly.

Comprehensive Opinions

Equally important, your opinion must be comprehensive. Having identified the issues, you must clearly articulate your opinions about them. Where expert reports are exchanged, failure to recite your opinion about each issue in your report may preclude you from offering such opinion at trial. Such a result will be damaging to the defense. Although the written report format may limit the detail you can comfortably provide, you certainly must explain each opinion thoroughly enough that the plaintiff's lawyer at trial cannot claim that your testimony is a "surprise".

Opinion Foundation

You must appreciate that the strength of an opinion is dependant upon the facts on which it is based. Offering opinions without a factual foundation is problematic. If all the facts necessary to support an opinion do not exist, reciting the opinion is counterproductive. Both you and your report will be discredited. Remember that theoretical ideals do little to enhance the practical role you were retained to fulfill. Ultimately, you will not be permitted to testify in court as an expert if your opinions are devoid of a factual underpinning. Such expert commentary is oftentimes termed "net opinion" and judges are careful to insulate juries from hearing testimony of this type. When writing your report, therefore, avoid offering opinions for which no factual support exists, no matter how interesting or compelling the issue may be.

Causation

It is not enough as a plaintiff to prove that a defendant deviated from the accepted standard of care. A plaintiff's ultimate success requires evidence that the defendant's negligence caused, contributed to, exacerbated or increased the risk of some injury or damage, that is, evidence of causation. Typically, the opinion testimony of an expert witness serves that purpose. Conversely, a defense expert retained to address the liability issue will normally be expected to comment about causation unless expressly advised by counsel not to do so or if the causation question requires comment by an expert in a different discipline. If you have been retained to address both the liability and causation issues, completely analyze both questions and, if required by the jurisdiction in which the case is venued, make certain that your report addresses both issues. Again, if you fail to include an opinion as to causation in your report, you will likely be precluded from offering it at trial. In other words, be complete.

Overreaching

This potential pitfall is more frequently found in a plaintiff's expert report than in that prepared by a defense expert.

However, the temptation to overreach crosses party lines. It is axiomatic that an expert practicing in a certain discipline should limit his opinions to that discipline or at least to treatment with which he has some experience.

In New Jersey, overreaching should not occur simply because current law requires, with rare exception, that the liability expert practice or teach in the same field as the defendant. However, in jurisdictions where such overreaching is not precluded, the following comments may prove helpful. By way of example, a gastroenterologist should typically not remark about the care provided by a general internist defendant even though gastroenterology is a subspecialty of internal medicine, unless of course the gastroenterologist provides general internal medicine care to patients as well. Decline to serve as the only expert in a case involving multiple defendants represented by the retaining defense attorney unless the defendants practice the same specialty. Instead, recommend to retaining counsel that he consider using multiple experts.

Of course, in certain jurisdictions, an exception to this rule exists. If in my internal medicine example, there are two defendants—one an internist and one a gastroenterologist—defense counsel might be permitted to utilize the expert services of a general internist so long as he provides gastroenterology care to his patients as part of his practice. In this situation, if the internist, based upon education, training and experience, has the requisite knowledge to comfortably and credibly offer opinions about the standard of care applicable to the treatment provided by the gastroenterologist, the internist could well serve as the single expert.

Again, in jurisdictions that embrace this exception, another example is illustrative. In a matter involving claims of malpractice against defendants in the fields of radiology and neurosurgery, arising out of the alleged improper interpretation of a CT scan of the head by the radiologist and negligent surgery by the neurosurgeon, a single neurosurgery expert would not be inappropriate so long as the neurosurgeon has experience

(as most do) in reading CT scans of the head and can convincingly address the claim that the radiologist's interpretation represented a departure from the accepted standard of care. Yet,
even if permissible, the better approach is to have a neurosurgery expert address the conduct of the defendant neurosurgeon and a radiologist help defend the defendant radiologist's
CT scan interpretation. Write about what you know or have
the capacity to know.

Attorney Summaries

Occasionally, as noted above, retaining attorneys will furnish you with a written summary of the salient facts. No
attorney expects that the expert will use the summary to the
exclusion of the primary documents upon which the summary is based. It typically is intended to serve as a thumb-
nail sketch of the relevant events, not a substitute for the
source materials you have been hired to review and analyze.
Once you have read the file materials, you may learn that
the summary is accurate—most are. On the other hand, you
may find that the summary is somewhat skewed in favor
of the party on whose behalf it has been drafted. To avoid
being influenced by the occasional inaccurate summary, do
not utilize it in formulating your opinions or in preparing
your report.

Items Reviewed

As previously mentioned, the initial section of your report
should list the materials furnished by counsel for your review.
Frequently, the number of items supplied is considerable. It is
important that you make certain that your report is accurate
in its recitation of those materials. This may seem like a "no
brainer", but I must tell you that there are occasions when the
expert report omits items that I believe have been supplied.
Although the omission typically is the result of an oversight or

a typographical error, my immediate concern is that the expert may have neglected to consider something in his assessment of the case or that a document that should have been forwarded to the expert was not. In order to avoid confusion, care should be taken to ensure that the list of materials is correct and complete.

Factual Accuracy

Another example of what might otherwise be the result of a simple oversight or typographical error is the mistaken reporting of basic numerical facts in the expert report. If it occurs at all, it usually happens in the discussion of dates, laboratory values and medical test results. Of course, if such errors reflect a failure to accurately glean critical facts upon which opinions are based, the ultimate result will likely be a flawed opinion. If, however, the errors are the result of careless keyboarding or proofreading, the end product may not be affected, but you will, nonetheless, appear sloppy or inattentive. Either way, attention to detail will avoid such mistakes. Of course, once received, the retaining attorney should carefully read your report and identify typos and other drafting errors. Expect that they will be brought to your attention.

Chapter 6

The Deposition

In jurisdictions like New Jersey, depositions of malpractice experts are routinely conducted. In many respects, the deposition serves as a precursor to the expert's trial appearance and can provide both information and insight to the examining attorney as well as the testifying expert. Depositions are verbal question and answer sessions conducted by adverse counsel, typically after all expert reports have been exchanged. They afford the opposing lawyer an opportunity to explore the expert's credentials and opinions. All attorneys involved in the matter are commonly present and entitled to conduct examination.

Location

Depositions historically have been taken either at the expert's office or at the office of the retaining lawyer. In some jurisdictions, a court reporter's office might be the location. Unless inconvenience is a major consideration because of the distance between your office and that of retaining counsel or because of your patient schedule, your deposition should be taken at the office of the retaining lawyer. The "sanitized" conference room of retaining counsel is preferable to the private office of an expert for the following reasons.

Since most practitioners' private offices have texts on shelves in plain view that the expert has gathered over the years, counsel may question the expert at deposition about relevant publications on those shelves. If any of the material in the expert's library is later found by the adverse attorney to contain statements inconsistent with the expert's opinion, it may be identified and used against the expert at trial.

Similarly, office waiting rooms often have brochures and pamphlets on display, which opposing attorneys might take and identify as items to be used at trial. Again, if any of this material, which you provide to your patients, contains information contrary to your report or deposition testimony, adverse counsel may use this fact to impeach you at trial. On balance, the convenience of scheduling the deposition at your office may be worth sacrificing in order to avoid potential problems created solely by the locale of the deposition.

Currently, the location of depositions has been impacted by COVID-19. Almost all depositions, including those of experts, are conducted remotely where the attorneys, the expert witness and the court reporter are all in separate locations. That said, the process remains the same. At some point, it is expected that in-person depositions will resume.

Fees

The fees associated with expert depositions are discretionary within reason. Time devoted to the deposition is properly and typically billed on the basis of an hourly fee schedule. Although discussed in an earlier section, it bears repeating that the customary hourly fee depending on the specialty of the expert ranges from $500 to $750. Some experts prefer to charge a flat rate, which also is generally acceptable so long as the total deposition fee when computed on an hourly basis at the conclusion of the deposition falls within this range. Reasonable fees for travel time to and from the deposition will be the responsibility of either the examining attorney or the retaining attorney as determined by the jurisdiction's court rules. Time devoted to deposition preparation and/or a pre-deposition meeting with retaining counsel will not be the responsibility of the attorney conducting the deposition. Reasonable hourly or flat fees for such effort are properly charged to the retaining lawyer.

Although some experts may insist on being paid by adverse counsel immediately upon the conclusion of the deposition, this is not customary. However, if receiving immediate payment is critical, inform retaining counsel of this requirement well in advance of the deposition date. Otherwise, generate a bill after the deposition and supply it to the retaining lawyer, who will then forward it to adverse counsel for payment.

Transcript

Testimony of the expert is given under oath and is recorded by a certified court reporter or stenographer hired by the attorney conducting the deposition. After the deposition, the expert's sworn testimony is transcribed by the court reporter and a transcript is prepared and usually furnished to all counsel within two to four weeks of the deposition. The retaining attorney should supply a copy of the transcript to you. If one is not received within 60 days of the deposition, contact retaining counsel and request a copy. Some but not all jurisdictions require that the transcript be read and signed by the witness.

Upon receipt of the deposition transcript, regardless of the local rules, take the time to read, not skim, the transcript. Make certain that the questions and your answers have been accurately recorded. Although court reporters are professionals and quite precise in their effort, the subject matter of a malpractice expert's deposition is highly technical and terminology employed by an expert witness may be foreign to even the most experienced of court reporters. Accordingly, the possibility exists that a mistake in recording can be made. Rapid speech or soft tones may also cause an error by the reporter, as can the circumstance where the questioner and the witness are speaking at the same time.

Inasmuch as a defendant's case may rise or fall on the testimony of the liability expert, and given the fact that deposition testimony can be used to impeach the expert at trial, it is essential that the deposition be accurately recorded. An unrecognized court reporter error that significantly alters an expert's testimony at deposition might be used against the expert at trial.

If you believe that the transcript contains an error, alert the retaining attorney as soon as possible. Counsel will then inform the court reporter, who is duty-bound to correct any transcription errors. Since court reporting equipment typically has voice-recording capability, confirming the accuracy of a stenographically recorded response can be readily accomplished.

Of course, actual testimony cannot be changed simply because you don't like your answer or the way a response reads. To prevent errors of this type, it is strongly recommended that you choose your words carefully and answer deliberately.

Purpose

The deposition allows the adverse attorney to inquire into the credentials of the expert and to explore the opinions held by that expert. It can be a relatively short or exceedingly protracted proceeding. The length of the deposition depends on several factors, including the content of the expert's Curriculum Vitae (CV), the number of defendants, the nature of the plaintiff's medical history, the complexity of the issues, the examining attorney's familiarity with the subject matter, the examining attorney's knowledge of the expert (as a result of the expert's participation in other matters), the length of the expert report, the number of opinions offered by the expert, the experience of the expert witness and the style of the examining lawyer or lawyers. Although a typical deposition may consume three hours, there are exceptions.

The deposition may be used both to gain a better understanding of the expert and the expert's opinions and to elicit testimony that may be valuable to the attorney taking the deposition. Although the examination may appear "exploratory", adverse counsel is probing for weaknesses or soft spots in the expert's opinions and will attempt to gain concessions from the expert. Experienced attorneys know that despite the conviction with which opinions appear to be held, carefully crafted deposition questions may cause the expert to reveal opinions favorable to the questioning attorney's client or to equivocate on certain pivotal issues.

It is expected that you will support at deposition previously articulated opinions. Do not cave. But also be reasonable. Indeed, reasonableness is the touchstone at deposition (and at trial). Your opinions should be reflective of the general notion that your practice area is not an exact science. You should be prepared to offer opinions based on probability. Of course, where an opinion can be stated with certainty, do so. But always recognize that in all but the rarest of circumstances, the opposite of the proposition you espouse on a given issue may be possible. What is not recommended, however, is to feign reasonableness by testifying that "anything is possible". This statement is absurd on its face and blatantly unsupportable. Expect that capable adverse counsel will use it against you at trial.

It is critical that you not answer any question that you do not understand. Instead, advise the examining attorney that the question is unclear and he will be required to clarify the question. No one can force you to respond to confusing or incomprehensible examination. Do not guess and avoid speculating. Do not offer information or opinions that are not requested. However, answer questions fully. If you provide

reasons in support of an opinion at trial that are not provided at deposition, this fact may be used against you at trial.

Although retaining counsel will be with you at the deposition, he is not your attorney. He is the lawyer for the defendant. Consequently, he can do little to "protect" you at the
deposition. Nor should he have to. Objections may be posed
by retaining counsel (or counsel for co-defendants where they
exist) to improperly formed questions. But, generally speaking, retaining counsel cannot force the examining attorney to
withdraw or rephrase a question. The rules governing attorney conduct and the degree to which counsel can "run interference" for you at deposition vary from state to state. However,
all jurisdictions expect that counsel will behave fairly at the
deposition, which necessarily dictates that the examination of
the expert will proceed without inappropriate objections by
retaining counsel.

Attire

Where permitted by local court rule, depositions of experts
may be video-recorded by adverse counsel and used at trial,
where appropriate. You should dress for the occasion. As
stated in an early section, your appearance is important to a
successful trial presentation. It is no less important at deposition, especially where the event is video-recorded. Even
absent recording, a positive physical appearance will serve to
impress. Accordingly, follow the rules of proper attire I discussed earlier.

Deposition Preparation

I have already stressed the importance of preparation as a
general proposition in the context of expert work. Indeed,

"anything worth doing, is worth doing right". The deposition is no exception, and in those venues where expert depositions are permitted, the expert deposition is a critical proceeding. It may prove to be pivotal in the defense of a malpractice action. It is the first opportunity the plaintiff's attorney has to pose questions and determine the effectiveness of the defense expert as a potential trial witness. It also represents an opportunity for the expert to get a sense of the style and demeanor of the attorney who may also be the cross-examining attorney at trial. In sum, the deposition serves as a forum for both the examiner and the examinee to "size-up" the opposition. Given the significance of the deposition, it is necessary that the expert devote sufficient effort to preparation.

The amount of time that likely will elapse between the initial review of documents and the deposition cannot be reliably predicted. It may be as short as a few weeks or as long as several months or even years. Although you may have been quite familiar with the factual details when you first examined the documents, your recollection of those details will fade with time. Thus, you should reacquaint yourself with the materials upon which you first based your opinions and with any additional materials received after your report was prepared. Do not rely on your memory alone. Refresh yourself well in advance of the deposition—not at the deposition. Otherwise, you will appear disorganized, unprofessional and less than fully competent. Also, you risk providing erroneous or ill-considered testimony that will be used to impeach you at trial.

Preparation also includes reviewing the salient facts and issues with the retaining attorney in a pre-deposition meeting. Although such sessions are typically less than two hours in length and may occur immediately prior to the deposition, the complexity of the matter may warrant a longer meeting and/or scheduling the pre-deposition meeting on a separate day prior to the actual deposition date.

Engage in a frank exchange of thoughts with defense counsel about the key documents and their content. Always make
certain that you have been supplied all the materials available for expert review, including but not limited to reports,
supplemental reports and depositions of other experts. To the
extent that information received after you initially reported
your opinions impacts those opinions, it is essential that you
disclose in sufficient detail the manner in which your opinions
have been affected. Materials that serve to bolster concepts
should be the subject of conversation, as should documents
that damage previously held opinions. Never fail to reveal to
defense counsel before the deposition newly discovered information that you know or should know will hurt the defendant
on whose behalf you have been retained. "Surprise" deposition testimony of this type is never appreciated by the retaining attorney. Should your lack of preparation or disclosure be
the cause, the damage done to the case (and your reputation)
may prove irreparable.

At the pre-deposition meeting, always invite discussion of the
issues and "problems" that might be expected at the deposition.
Inquire about expected lines of questioning and discuss how
you anticipate responding. It also is recommended that key portions of discovery, including the deposition testimony of parties,
nonparty witnesses and other experts, be reviewed to the extent
that such discovery may be important to an issue likely to be
raised at your deposition.

In the end, no one expects you to have a flawless memory
of all the minute details. You are expected, however, to have
a working knowledge of the important facts and their sources.
By no means should you have a cavalier attitude about the significance of the deposition. Appreciate your role at the deposition and prepare with the same degree of intensity as if you
were appearing at trial. Realize that any lapse will be exploited
by opposing counsel at trial. Conversely, a strong performance
at deposition may dissuade adverse counsel from aggressively
attacking you at trial.

Available Documents

To the extent that your opinions are based upon a review of documents supplied to you by counsel, the retaining attorney might recommend that all of those documents be brought to the pre-deposition meeting and the deposition itself. If the materials are electronically stored, you may be asked to bring the thumb drive, disc and/or laptop. In this way, you will have available to you all the materials you reviewed. Suffice it to say, it is far better to have your file available to you in some form rather than to leave all or portions of it behind. Well in advance of the deposition, the plaintiff's attorney frequently will serve retaining counsel with a written request for your file materials and expect their production at the deposition. The retaining lawyer will alert you if this occurs and advise as to the documents the local rules require you to produce.

In some states, written or verbal communications between the expert and retaining counsel that constitute part of the "collaborative process" are privileged and therefore protected from inquiry by adverse counsel at deposition and/or trial. Frequently, emails, text messages and notes to and from the expert that explore strategy or that reflect the exchange of ideas are considered confidential and therefore need not be brought to the deposition. Other jurisdictions, however, consider every-thing supplied to the expert by retaining counsel or furnished to the retaining lawyer by the expert to be discoverable. That is, nothing is confidential. The retaining attorney should guide you about the rules in the jurisdiction where the matter is venued.

Areas of Examination

The deposition typically begins with a series of questions about your credentials. If your CV was previously supplied to retaining counsel with your report, as is often the case, defense counsel probably furnished it to adverse counsel with your report. As a result, the examining lawyer will have a "jumping off" point from which to begin questioning. The background portion of the deposition will be shortened because much of the information one might obtain by oral examination is contained in the CV. Expect that the attorney will ask you to confirm both that the CV is accurate and current. To the extent that the CV requires updating, you will be asked to verbally do so at the deposition.

Once your credentials are explored, you usually will be asked about your experience as a retained expert in legal matters generally and malpractice cases specifically. You will be asked to disclose the number of cases that you have received and accepted for review and the percentage breakdown between plaintiff and defense cases. Although you may not want to act as a plaintiff's malpractice expert, as your expert work develops, accepting an occasional plaintiff's case will enhance your credibility as a defense expert. A practitioner who is revealed as a defense expert exclusively loses some credibility. For this reason, defense attorneys might not regularly retain such an expert. Therefore, you should consider serving as a plaintiff's liability expert from time to time but only when the defendant's conduct clearly has violated a standard of care and has contributed to an alleged injury.

Expect to be questioned about various collateral matters. Also expect that your testimony about such matters might be used at trial to impair your credibility. The information might also serve as the basis for adverse counsel to conduct a secondary investigation of you in anticipation of your trial appearance. For example, you may be asked about the following: (1) your experience giving deposition or trial testimony; (2) how often you have worked with retaining counsel or other attorneys in that firm; (3) whether you ever have been retained by attorneys representing any other defendants in this matter; (4) your fee structure; (5) how often you advertise your services as an expert or list your name with agencies that provide names of experts to lawyers; (6) license suspensions or other

adverse regulatory action; (7) the loss, interruption or modifi-
cation of hospital privileges; (8) the percentage of professional
time you devote to expert work; (9) the percentage of your
total income derived from expert work and (10) your personal
experience as a defendant in malpractice cases.

You also may be asked about published texts in your
field which you consider to be "authoritative". If any such
acknowledged texts contain passages that are inconsistent with your opinions, adverse counsel might use them
in cross-examination of you at trial. You should always
be careful about identifying texts as authoritative for this
reason. I have seen experts resist identifying any text as
authoritative in part by stating that the information contained in a textbook, by definition, is outdated by the time
it's published. An expert might only be willing to testify that a text is a standard, useful or somewhat reliable
work making it difficult for adverse counsel to discredit
the expert's opinions with passages from that textbook.
Frequently, an expert will indicate that information found in
peer reviewed journal articles is more current and reliable.

The balance of the deposition will be devoted to an explo-
ration of your experience treating the condition which is
the subject of the case, the relevant facts and your substantive opinions about the matter. It is during this portion of
the deposition that the sufficiency of your preparation will
be tested, as will be your knowledge of the pertinent events
and the relative strength of your opinions. Expect to be
asked questions about the facts referenced in your report and
those you may have deliberately omitted. Keep in mind that
although you may have discussed in your report the facts you
deemed significant, counsel is entitled to inquire about other
germane facts found in the documents you were supplied but
that were not referenced in your report. To the extent that
you have a working knowledge of those facts, responding to
questions about them should not prove difficult. However, if
questions are asked about lesser-known facts or even those

that you might consider obscure, insist on being permitted to review the necessary materials before providing an answer. Here is where my earlier instruction to bring your file documents to the deposition will be appreciated. Of course, never guess in response to a question posed.

Usually, new opinions will not be offered at the deposition. Where adverse counsel has received your reports in advance of the deposition, it is expected that all of your pertinent opinions are recited in those writings. Generally speaking, surprising the examining lawyer with opinions never previously expressed is inappropriate. The expert report is intended to embody all of the material opinions of the expert, albeit in abbreviated fashion. While the expert is not expected to disclose new opinions during a deposition that could have been included in the report, the expert is permitted to offer opinions that reasonably flow from those opinions contained in the report.

There are times, though rare, when offering new opinions at deposition is unavoidable. For example, if newly identified documents are reviewed by an expert shortly before the deposition, new opinions prompted by that review might be properly offered at deposition. Further, if the examining attorney asks questions that naturally and necessarily require a response that incorporates a new opinion, the expert cannot be criticized for offering one.

Gratuitous Testimony

At deposition, the liability expert should limit his remarks to his area of expertise and should not comment on matters irrelevant to the opinion the expert was retained to provide.

If you are serving as a liability defense expert in a matter that involves multiple defendants who practice in different disciplines, you probably were retained to offer a liability opinion about a defendant who practices in your specialty.

Yet, as previously discussed, there may be jurisdictions that permit you to opine regarding treatment provided by a defendant who specializes in another discipline, because the treatment is part of your expertise as well, that is, there's an overlap between your specialty and that of the defendant. For example, both an orthopedic surgeon and a general diagnostic radiologist are competent to read orthopedic x-rays and a neurosurgeon and a neuroradiologist can both interpret CT scans of the brain.

However, in a matter involving multiple defendants, each one may be represented by different counsel and each attorney typically will retain a liability expert. Thus, there may be numerous defense experts in a given case. If you should be retained as the liability expert for one of the defendants, the scope of your critique will be limited to the conduct of that one defendant. Although you may conclude that the practitioner on whose behalf you have been retained and other defendants were not negligent, because you have not been hired to serve as an expert for the other defendants, you should confine your opinion to the defendant on whose behalf you were retained. Although it may be comforting to the defense as a whole that you find no fault in the acts of other defendants, your report should avoid commentary about them. Leave the defense of the other defendants to their attorneys and their liability experts (unless expressly advised otherwise by retaining counsel).

Similarly, at deposition, do not gratuitously offer remarks about the other defendants. Your focus should be the practitioner on whose behalf you have been retained. Expanding the scope of your opinions to encompass other defendants may prove problematic, especially if you practice outside their specialties, if your grasp of the facts as affects other defendants is not firm or if you offer comment which is not absolutely consistent with the opinions of the experts retained to aid in their defense. If you "stumble" in commenting about the other defendants, you likely will do more harm than good as concerns them and, in the process, will dilute the strength of the opinions you were retained to offer.

The exception occurs most often in matters where there is more than one defendant who practices in the same discipline and where each of the defendants was involved in the treatment of the same ongoing condition. I recall one such case that involved three orthopedic surgeon defendants, each of whom was involved in treating a non-displaced transverse fracture of the plaintiff's distal tibial shaft. Immediately following the plaintiff's injury, one of the physicians saw the plaintiff in a hospital emergency department, the second saw the plaintiff for follow-up treatment in the office for a series of visits and the third saw the plaintiff on a single occasion as the covering doctor for the second physician when he was on vacation. The plaintiff was treated non-surgically with casting in the emergency department by the on-call orthopedic surgeon and the subsequent orthopedic surgeons continued the same treatment plan.

I represented the covering orthopedic surgeon, and on his behalf, I retained an orthopedic surgeon as my expert. After he reviewed the file materials, he advised that my client did not deviate from the accepted standard of care and that based on his review of the facts, he believed that neither of the other two defendants had acted negligently. Since the lawyer who represented the other two doctors had retained an expert on their behalf, my expert drafted a report in which he only commented about my client. Before his deposition, however, I advised that if expressly asked at deposition about the other defendants, he could and should comment about their treatment. As expected, the plaintiff's attorney did inquire and my expert testified that none of the orthopedic surgeons had deviated from the accepted standard of care.

I advised my expert to provide this opinion for a number of reasons. First, the pitfalls that often exist in situations where an expert "overreaches" were not present here. All of the defendants practiced in the same discipline. The facts that applied to all the defendants were simple and easily grasped by my expert. Because each defendant followed the same treatment plan, the malpractice issues as to each defendant were the same, and my expert's response to the liability claims was utterly consistent with that of the expert retained on behalf of the other two defendants. In fact, under these circumstances, my expert's opinion was strengthened, not diluted, by the consistency of his thinking as applied to each of the defendants, all of whom followed a uniform treatment plan.

I am reminded of another matter in which I represented an obstetrician whose alleged malpractice resulted in the birth of a brain-damaged baby. The case involved an obstetrical patient who, having detected decreased fetal movement, had an office-based non-stress test, the results of which were not reassuring. She was then referred by her obstetrician to a hospital perinatal diagnostic testing center where the biophysical profile score unfortunately was a dismal two out of ten. The perinatologist at the hospital testing center referred the patient to the hospital's Labor and Delivery floor for observation and delivery. There, she was met by my client, the partner of the patient's primary obstetrician. After being assured by the perinatologist that an emergency cesarean section delivery was not necessarily required, my client left the hospital following notification of the nurses. Within minutes of his departure, the fetal monitoring strips indicated that the fetus' condition had deteriorated. Due to my client's absence from the hospital, another obstetrician delivered the baby, which had profound brain damage.

The other defendants were the patient's primary obstetrician and the hospital perinatologist. Each of these physicians had separate counsel and each retained a separate liability expert. I retained the services of a widely recognized perinatologist. After my expert completed his review of the relevant documents, he advised that my client had not departed from the accepted standard of care. He also believed that none of the other defendants had deviated. In his opinion, the outcome, though unfortunate, was not the result of anyone's malpractice. Although my expert had sufficient expertise to remark about the conduct of the patient's treating obstetrician and the hospital's perinatologist, I instructed him to limit his remarks to my client and his report was prepared accordingly. Similarly, at deposition, he confined his comments to the acts of my client alone.

Unlike the first example involving the tibial shaft fracture, here the facts were extremely complex, the role played by each of the defendant practitioners in the continuum of care was unique and the claims of malpractice were different as to each defendant. Moreover, my client was the primary target of the malpractice action, and it was essential to his defense that the expert devote his full attention to my client's conduct. It would not have aided my client if the retained expert gratuitously tried to assist the other defendants. In fact, given my client's position as the litigation's focus, it is likely that the co-defendants wanted to maintain their distance from my client and our expert.

Chapter 7

The Trial

Other than when a case settles or is dismissed, everything culminates in the trial. A successful trial outcome requires that each phase of the trial be carefully executed. One phase, indeed one of the most important and most powerful, involves the presentation of expert testimony.

Of course, COVID-19 has interrupted scheduled malpractice trials everywhere and upon their resumption, they may not immediately resemble the traditional process. Although the physical construct may be altered in the short term, the components of the trial and the participants will remain the same. The discussion below contemplates a traditional trial, but the concepts are universally applicable regardless of COVID-19's impact on tradition.

Fees

Fees associated with an expert's trial appearance have already been reviewed in detail. Most experts establish court appearance rates on a flat fee basis for either a half- or full-day appearance. Some experts charge hourly fees consistent with the schedule established for deposition testimony. In addition to time spent in court, and regardless of what the court appearance fee arrangement is, fees associated with trial preparation (including document review and conferences with retaining counsel) are typically charged on an hourly basis.

Pre-trial Preparation

It bears repeating that success as an expert requires adequate preparation. A quality expert report and strong deposition testimony are both based in large part upon sufficient preparation. A successful trial presentation is no exception and, in fact, depends largely upon the degree to which you prepare. I am convinced that in the long run, finesse and style will take you just so far as a trial witness. Whether a jury accepts your opinion depends on how well you articulate it, support it and defend it. To do those things, you must master the facts, issues and arguments. You must be prepared for the attacks on your position that will be made on cross-examination, often by a skilled, experienced lawyer who is being assisted by his or her expert. Without preparation, you stand little chance of succeeding at trial.

Preparation requires a willingness to devote significant time to rereading the relevant materials supplied to you when you rendered your initial opinion. It requires that you read or reread all relevant documents supplied to you after you furnished your initial opinion, including written discovery such as interrogatory answers and the deposition testimony of parties and nonparty witnesses. You must also read the reports and deposition testimony of all other experts. If professional journals or textbook excerpts have been identified, reread them and generally know their content. Make certain that you know the factual details of the case and be ready to discuss them in court. Should your preparation be lacking in this regard, you will undoubtedly falter, as will the defense you were retained to bolster.

If you have authored reports, reread them. If you have been deposed, read the transcript of your deposition. If an opinion you have offered is not supported by newly discovered facts, alert retaining counsel and discuss the manner in which the potential adverse impact of these facts can be softened. As previously discussed, you should bring file materials to the trial in electronical or paper form and have them in court in an organized fashion, unless directed otherwise by defense counsel.

Pre-trial and pre-testimony conferences with the retaining lawyer are absolutely essential. My preference is that my expert and I meet in person or virtually before the trial begins. At that time, I generally review my expert's opinions, identify and examine key documents, discuss potential pitfalls, address the opinions of adverse experts, review areas of anticipated direct examination and cross-examination, discuss the creation and use of trial aids and arrange the order of evidence presentation. You can expect that retaining counsel will initiate this meeting. At a minimum, the expert and counsel should speak about the case on the telephone before the trial begins.

In addition to the pre-trial meeting, I recommend a pre-testimony conference that can be conducted by telephone. As a defense attorney, I typically prefer this second preparation session to occur on the day or evening before the expert is scheduled to testify. By this point, the plaintiff's case has been fully presented, including the testimony of the plaintiff's expert or experts. The issues have been honed, and the documents used by the plaintiff at trial are now a matter of record. I then can focus my expert's attention on that which has already occurred at trial and advise him as to my assessment of the relative strengths and weaknesses of the plaintiff's case. I also am able to discuss the opinions of the plaintiff's expert as offered in court and critique the jury's outward reaction to those opinions. A review of specific questions I intend to pose at trial on direct examination and those I expect will be asked by adverse counsel is also part of this conference.

Understanding Your Environment

To the novice expert, the courtroom is foreign territory. As a tangible symbol of the law, the courtroom's trappings are largely based on tradition and are reflective of a palpable melding of custom and purpose.

Your effectiveness as an expert requires that you understand the environment in which you have been asked to perform. You must be comfortable in the courtroom and you must appear comfortable to the jury. An expert who seems ill at ease on the witness stand will be poorly received by jurors. Even the most solid expert opinion will seem less credible and less persuasive if the person delivering the opinion is unable to comfortably function in court.

In order to achieve some degree of comfort, you must understand the physical environment and the roles of the typical trial participants. Since you likely spend most of your time in a hospital or practice office where your comfort level is high, the courtroom will present a new challenge. Even if you do a fair amount of public speaking at conferences and lectures to colleagues, you still will be out of your element in court.

One recommended and highly effective way in which an inexperienced expert can combat this problem is to spend time in the courtroom before testifying. I suggest that if you are not the first witness of the trial day, you arrive at least 30–60 minutes early. Sit in court and watch the proceedings. Learn the behavioral tendencies of the various "players" in the trial. Appreciate the dynamics of the relationship between and among the human components of the trial—the judge (sometimes referred to as "the court"), the jury, the plaintiff's attorney, the defense attorney, the plaintiff, the defendant, the court officer (or bailiff), the court clerk and occasionally the judge's law clerk. Watch the jurors and their reaction to trial events—attorney questions, witness answers, objections by counsel, the judge's rulings, physical movement by attorneys and witnesses and the use of trial aids and exhibits. If you are offered this opportunity, seize it. You will be amazed at how your anxiety level will decrease.

Although I am a proponent of this exercise, I must caution you that in some situations, the trial judge will not permit expert witnesses to sit in court and observe the testimony of other witnesses. At times, the trial judge, prompted by a request from counsel, will direct that expert witnesses be sequestered outside the courtroom until the expert actually testifies. Therefore, if you plan to appear early, ask retaining counsel if you will be permitted to sit in court prior to testifying.

Trial Sequence

In addition to appreciating the physical characteristics of the courtroom and the role of each participant, you should also understand how a trial proceeds and some of the more general "rules" of behavior in court.

The trial begins with a brief statement by the judge to the panel of prospective jurors about that nature of the case, the allegations and the defenses. The attorneys are then introduced and each attorney introduces his or her client and identifies the anticipated trial witnesses. The prospective jurors provide information about themselves in open court in response to questions posed by the judge and/or counsel. The trial judge will excuse certain individuals from service "for cause", that is, due to personal experiences, familiarity with the parties, attorneys or witnesses, financial hardship, medical reasons, language difficulties, a pre-arranged vacation, work requirements or personal/family obligations. The court can excuse an infinite number of jurors "for cause". Each of the attorneys may excuse from service certain of the jurors, as well. Generally, an attorney can exercise a "peremptory" challenge and excuse a prospective juror for an undisclosed reason consistent with prevailing law without articulating the reason. However, the presumption is that the juror has identified something in his or her personal background or has displayed a characteristic that the attorney believes might reasonably suggest a bias either against his client or in favor of the adverse party. Absent exceptional circumstances, each attorney is given a fixed number of peremptory jury challenges. Once those challenges are exhausted, counsel cannot seek to eliminate any further prospective jurors without cause.

Typically, after jury selection and preliminary remarks or instructions by the trial judge, the substantive trial begins with an opening statement by the plaintiff's attorney (whose seat at counsel table is closest to the jury box) followed by the opening statement of the defendant's lawyer (whose seat at counsel table is furthest from the jury box). If the trial involves multiple defendants, the sequence of defense opening statements will follow the order in which the various defendants have been named in the Complaint. Witnesses and evidence will then be presented by the plaintiff's attorney, at the conclusion of which, the plaintiff will "rest". The defense case is then presented with witnesses and other evidence. Again, if there are multiple defendants, each defendant presents his or her case in the same order as opening statements. Each defendant will "rest" at the conclusion of that defendant's presentation of witnesses and evidence. In rare instances, the plaintiff may present "rebuttal" evidence in response to unanticipated critical evidence offered by the defense.

After presentation of all evidence, a summation or closing argument will be offered by each attorney. The sequence will be the opposite of the opening statements. Opening and closing remarks by the lawyers are not evidence, and the jury is so advised by the trial judge. The court then instructs the jurors as to the law that applies to the case, called the "Jury Charge". The jury is obligated during deliberations to apply the law recited by the trial judge during the Jury Charge to the facts as it finds existed based on the evidence. Following deliberations in the jury room (which may take minutes or days), the jury records its decision on a Jury Verdict Sheet and then returns to the courtroom to verbally announce its verdict in open court to the judge, the parties and their counsel.

A Jury Verdict Sheet in a very basic malpractice case with issues of liability, causation and damages may look like this sample:

VERDICT SHEET

_____ v._____

Docket No. xxxxx

1. Did the defendant deviate from the accepted standard of care in the treatment of the plaintiff?

Yes_____ No_____

If your answer to question 1 is yes, proceed to question 2. If your answer to question 1 is no, cease your deliberations and return your verdict.

2. Was the defendant's deviation from the accepted standard of care a proximate cause of the plaintiff's injuries and damages?

Yes_____ No_____

If your answer to question 2 is yes, proceed to question 3. If your answer to question 2 is no, cease your deliberations and return your verdict.

3. What amount of money would fairly and reasonably compensate the plaintiff for pain, suffering, disability, impairment and loss of enjoyment of life?

Amount_____

Agree_____ Disagree_____

Affirmative answers to both the first and second questions establish that the defendant was negligent and that such negligence
was a substantial cause of the injuries and damages alleged.
The jury must then decide the amount of money to which the
plaintiff is entitled. A negative response to either the first or
second question will result in a verdict in favor of the defendant.
A positive response to the first question alone is insufficient to
return a verdict for the plaintiff. In order for the defendant to be
found liable, the jury must determine that the defendant acted
negligently and that the negligent conduct was a proximate
cause of the plaintiff's alleged injuries and damages. A "proximate cause" is often defined as a cause that set other causes in
motion and was a substantial factor in bringing about the alleged
injury. It is an event which naturally and probably led to and
might have been expected to produce the alleged result.

Of course, a more complex case involving additional
issues such as informed consent, aggravation of a pre-existing
medical condition, comparative negligence or mitigation of
damages, or which includes a plaintiff's spouse or multiple
defendants will complicate the proofs at trial and increase the
number of questions on the Jury Verdict Sheet.

In jurisdictions like New Jersey, eight jurors are usually
selected at the beginning of a civil trial. At the trial's conclusion, immediately after the Jury Charge, two of the eight are
randomly selected as alternates and the remaining six jurors
will deliberate. Of course, if one or two jurors are excused
during the trial due to illness or inability to serve for any other
reason, the trial judge may only need to excuse one juror or
perhaps no one before deliberations begin. If a deliberating
juror suddenly is unable to participate, one of the alternates
will take that juror's place.

In lengthy trials, a judge may be inclined to allow all eight
jurors to deliberate. Usually, such thinking is prompted by the
court's belief that jurors who participate in a protracted trial
should not be arbitrarily precluded from participating in the deliberations. However, this is only allowed if all the parties agree.

Typically, a verdict in a civil case need not be unanimous, no matter the number of jurors. Rather, with a requisite six-member jury, a question on a Jury Verdict Sheet is considered answered if at least five of the six jurors provide the same response. Importantly, the same five jurors need not agree as to each question. If all eight jurors deliberate, a Jury Verdict Sheet question is answered if at least seven jurors agree.

Upon announcement of the jury's verdict in open court, a judgment is entered in favor of the prevailing party and the trial phase is formally over. Motions may thereafter follow (almost always by the losing party), and an appeal may be filed. Usually, however, the end of the trial is the end of the malpractice lawsuit.

Intra-trial Events

During trial, counsel will often address the court using rather formal language intended to convey a sense of respect properly due the trial judge. It is expected that counsel also will be addressed by the court with appropriate respect. Witnesses are also to be treated with respect by examining counsel. And of course, the jury is deserving of the respect of all trial participants.

When it is necessary, address the trial judge as "Your Honor". Although you may invoke the more casual term "Judge", use it less frequently than "Your Honor". Refer to retaining and examining counsel as "Mr. _____" or "Ms. _____" or "Counsel". Unless instructed otherwise by the retaining lawyer, parties should be referred to as "Mr. _____", "Ms. _____" or "Dr. _____".

The trial judge may interrupt your response to a question at any time. If this should happen, stop talking and defer to the court and its need to comment. If your testimony is interrupted by a remark from either counsel (typically an

objection), stop and allow counsel to complete his or her statement and await instruction from the court or examining counsel as to if or how you may proceed.

A typical and repeated occurrence during a trial is the sidebar conference. Over time, it serves as a source of annoyance
and frustration to witnesses and jurors alike. A "sidebar" conference is a mini meeting between the trial judge and counsel.
It takes place alongside the judge's bench opposite the witness
stand and may be convened at the direction of the trial judge
or at the request of one of the attorneys. The remarks by the
trial judge and counsel are not intended for witness or jury
consumption. Consequently, voices must be kept in low tones
so as to minimize the possibility that a witness or a juror may
overhear the discussion. A sidebar often occurs in response
to an objection by one of the lawyers to a question or as a
result of testimony elicited from a witness. In such instance,
the topic of discussion is one that involves issues of law and/
or evidence. Procedural or scheduling matters may also be
addressed at sidebar.

Although exceptions exist, most sidebars are brief, usually
lasting from 30 seconds to five minutes. If, after the sidebar
begins, it appears to the trial judge that the conference will
consume significantly more time, the court may direct the jury
to return to the jury room, and the witness may be asked by
the judge to temporarily leave the courtroom. Excusing the
jurors and the witness protects them from overhearing the
sidebar. Possibly prejudicial comments by counsel which jurors
and perhaps witnesses overhear may be the basis for a mistrial
and the subsequent need to start the trial process anew at a
later date with a new jury.

At the conclusion of the sidebar, the trial judge will typically advise the jury as to the court's ruling in response to the
objection of counsel or otherwise remark to the extent necessary. If the ruling impacts you as the trial witness, an instruction from the court will be offered. In such instance, comply
with the judge's direction and, if appropriate, respectfully

acknowledge the judge's comments with a simple "Yes, Your Honor" or similar response.

Of course, multiple sidebar conferences during your testimony can disrupt your presentation and make it less effective. In fact, sidebars necessitated by adverse counsel's constant objections may be part of a deliberate effort to rattle you. No matter how frustrating, don't let the interruptions "throw you". Maintain your composure and, when permitted by the trial judge to continue, do so smoothly. Focus on the substance of your testimony and ignore adverse counsel's maneuvers.

Also potentially problematic is the "dead time" created by the sidebar. While the sidebar conference takes place, you may be on the witness stand in front of the jury. Members of the jury likely are watching you, trying to "size you up". Don't squirm in your seat, tug at your collar or nervously shuffle the papers before you. Although you may not talk to the jury, the interlude presents an opportunity to enhance your rapport with the jury. Instead of looking away from the jury, you may make brief eye contact with the jurors. Look their way in a relaxed, easy and confident fashion.

Also, be aware that the judge may question you during a trial. Such questioning typically is infrequent and there is no way to predict whether or when it will occur. Customarily, the court poses queries when the judge feels that those asked by the attorneys do not fully explore a significant issue. A judge may also question a witness where the testimony is confusing, meandering or evasive (unintentionally or deliberately). Although many judges are reluctant to assume the role of lawyer, it is the court's duty to ensure that the evidence is fairly and completely presented to the jury. To that end, therefore, judges at times inject themselves into the examination process in order to assist the jury in its fact-finding effort. Accordingly, you must be prepared to field court-initiated questions, which are typically direct and pointed. Needless to say, answer them forthrightly. Judges have far less tolerance than do attorneys for answers that are circuitous or confusing. Even if the judge appears to incorporate the position of the opposing party in the questions posed or to adopt an adversarial tone, respond with the requisite respect and avoid being combative.

Finally, in some states, jurors are permitted to question witnesses after the attorneys complete their examination. Typically, jury questions are handwritten by jurors and then reviewed by the trial judge and counsel. They may be slightly modified by the judge where appropriate and then presented verbally to the witness by the judge. Respond with the same care as you would in answering questions posed by counsel or the court.

Understanding Your Role

As an expert witness, you are one of the most impactful and powerful "players" in the trial. You are not, however, the director. You serve at the behest of the retaining attorney. Further, the courtroom is the domain of the trial judge. Your performance is limited by rules known by the attorneys and enforced by the judge. It is not your prerogative to control any aspect of the trial other than your testimony. Accept direction from questioning counsel and respond to instruction offered by the trial judge.

Also, you may not control the date and time of your courtroom appearance. Although retaining counsel will work with you and try to accommodate your schedule, satisfying requests for specific appearance dates and times is often impossible. As you must appreciate, the trial is stressful for everyone, including counsel, and scheduling witnesses is often complicated.

The trial is fluid. Witness scheduling at the outset is typically based on expectations of how quickly (or slowly) the trial will progress. Those expectations often must be revised as the trial unfolds. Scheduling is affected by numerous factors over which counsel has little or no control, such as: (1) the length of jury selection; (2) obligations of the judge that disrupt the trial; (3) the length of witness testimony; (4) court recesses; (5) unanticipated protracted legal arguments; (6) the frequency and duration of sidebar conferences; and (7) miscellaneous "down time". Also, infrequently, an unanticipated trial development prompts a change in trial strategy and an attorney may determine that a scheduled witness may not be needed, that a witness the attorney initially did not plan to call becomes necessary or that the anticipated order in which witnesses were to be presented must change.

Lawyers recognize that experts are not just "standing by" waiting to testify and that practice constraints limit flexibility. However, any effort expended by the expert to accommodate the attorney's view of when the expert's appearance will be most effective will be appreciated.

The liability defense expert usually is one of the last witnesses to appear for a defendant. If the liability expert is also offering opinions on causation or damages, it makes sense to present such evidence at or near the end of the defendant's proofs where it will have the most impact.

As a defense attorney, I rarely put any of my experts on the stand before the testimony of my client or that of nonparty defense witnesses. I firmly believe that the expert typically is the strength of my client's case, and I can optimize the expert's effectiveness by having the expert testify last. Since the expert's opinions are based upon the facts, it's logical to present the fact witnesses, including the defendant practitioner, before presenting the expert. The expert can utilize the facts offered by earlier witnesses in support of the expert's opinions. Additionally, the expert's testimony likely will be remembered by the jury and therefore have the greatest impact on the trial outcome if heard as close to jury deliberations as possible. Of course, there may be times, albeit few, when as a result of circumstances dictated by events over which I have no control, I am unable to conclude my presentation with the expert witness. Those circumstances should not include, however, the intractability of the expert over appearance scheduling.

Also understand that you are not an advocate for the defendant on whose behalf you have been retained. That is the role of defense counsel. You were initially hired to review the case as a neutral, dispassionate, third party for purposes of offering an independent opinion. That has not changed just because you are now in court.

Courtroom Demeanor

Your role as a liability expert, as you now can understand, dictates in large measure your demeanor in court. Identified and presented by retaining counsel as a highly credentialed, experienced and knowledgeable practitioner in your field, you likely will be well-received by the jury for the first few minutes of your opinion testimony. Typically, jurors will listen with a relatively open mind, and if you capture their attention with the logic of your thoughts and the certainty of your opinions, that elusive yet essential goal of jury acceptance may be yours.

However, though rare, there are trial events that can be so devastating that they taint a litigant's case and all associated with it. By way of example, I once defended a podiatrist whom the plaintiff alleged had botched bunion surgery. At the time of the procedure, the plaintiff was employed as a housekeeper. She maintained that as a result of the malpractice, she could no longer tolerate the physical demands of housecleaning. She claimed, therefore, that she was forced to resign her position with a family on whose behalf she had worked for years. During the discovery period, the plaintiff remained unemployed and advanced the position that the operated foot was in such bad shape that she could not work. Suspicious of her claims, I retained a private investigator to conduct video surveillance of the plaintiff, and we struck gold.

My investigator obtained footage of the plaintiff engaging in activities of daily living without any obvious problems— no limp, no special footgear, no devices to aid in walking, no difficulty going up and down stairs and no problem digging with a shovel in her yard. But the best piece of recorded surveillance revealed that this unemployed housekeeper could indeed do housework. Quite fortuitously, my investigator caught her cleaning houses with a crew of two other women. Amazingly, the plaintiff was video-recorded inside a home standing in a front room cleaning a large picture window, the window sill and the framed photographs sitting on the sill. Nonetheless, the plaintiff testified under oath at deposition that she could not perform any house cleaning duties at all and that she did not clean homes with the two other women who were surveilled.

Nice, right? But, you must be thinking, "What does this have to do with expert testimony?" Simply this: During my opening statement, I advised the jury that notwithstanding the plaintiff's claimed disability and inability to work, I intended to present surveillance video which unequivocally demonstrated otherwise. What the jury would see was reviewed in detail. I established the groundwork for the portrayal of the plaintiff as a malingerer, a fabricator and a fraud. I wanted a certain reaction from the jury during my opening, and I got it. From that point forward, everything the plaintiff and her attorney did and said during that trial was viewed with skepticism. Although her well-rehearsed direct testimony was relatively flawless, the plaintiff's testimony in response to cross-examination was anything but. The plaintiff claimed that she neither spoke nor understood English and so she testified with the aid of a translator. As the plaintiff got caught up in my questioning, however, she began to answer before the interpreter finished translating my English and at times did so without waiting for even one word to be translated. The plaintiff also began answering my questions in English rather than in her native tongue. Suffice it to say, the jury quickly saw the plaintiff for what she was.

Interesting also was the plaintiff's lawyer's decision to play the surveillance video during his client's testimony. Although

I later presented the recorded surveillance with the testimony of my private investigator as part of the defense case, the plaintiff's attorney's decision to have the jury view the surveillance early in the trial was a bold but ineffective maneuver. It was clear to me that he was hoping to diffuse the power of the surveillance video by showing it during his client's direct testimony, giving her an opportunity to explain away what everyone saw. The strategy backfired. Not only was the plaintiff completely unbelievable in her testimony about the recorded surveillance, but the jury now was able to see this evidence twice and earlier in the trial than it normally occurs.

Keep in mind that the plaintiff's testimony and the viewing of the recorded surveillance both occurred before the plaintiff's expert ever got on the stand. Imagine now, against this backdrop, the appearance of the plaintiff's expert. No matter how qualified, how experienced, how knowledgeable or how competent, that expert stood no chance of succeeding. The plaintiff's case was so badly damaged that there was nothing the plaintiff's expert could do or say that would change the jury's suspicion of the plaintiff's claims.

The impact of successful surveillance was again demonstrated in another malpractice trial where the plaintiff claimed depth perception and balance issues as a result of impaired vision in one eye following the defendant's strabismus surgery. No matter the strength of the plaintiff's expert's trial testimony, the plaintiff's case was significantly damaged when the jury saw surveillance video of plaintiff capably walking up and down stairs at her local gym without holding the handrail. The surveillance footage also revealed plaintiff in a spinning class. Never once did plaintiff appear to lose her balance. Even better, the jury watched in apparent amazement as plaintiff took a rather advanced yoga class where she had absolutely no problem assuming a series of poses again without losing her balance.

Surveillance at the local food market revealed that the plaintiff was able to push a cart and shop for items in various departments without bumping into anyone or anything.

This clip was inconsistent with the plaintiff's boyfriend's trial testimony that because plaintiff was prone to bumping her shopping cart into people and objects, he always accompanied her so he could maneuver her cart. He was nowhere to be found in the video.

No matter how capable the plaintiff's liability expert, the surveillance video again proved too compelling for any expert to overcome.

However, assuming no such unusual development, your demeanor will influence the jury. Therefore, certain of the intangibles that comprise demeanor are worth reviewing.

Confidence is critical and cannot be underestimated. However, there is a fine line between confidence and arrogance. Given lay tendencies to view physicians in the real world as arrogant, it is not surprising that jurors might perceive experts with the same jaundiced eye. Consequently, when testifying, do so with confidence but always guard against tripping on the line that divides confidence and arrogance.

In my view, a confident expert is one who testifies with a certain degree of passion. By that, I am not endorsing raised tones or table pounding. I am simply suggesting that, where appropriate, incorporate some emotion into your testimony. Don't be afraid to be passionate about your opinions. You should convey conviction that you are right and that the defendant acted properly.

Of course, the jury's perception of you as a confident witness may be the result in part of your actions even when you are not actually speaking. Given the fact that the jury will be watching you throughout your time on the witness stand, never do anything that will be ill-received. Let me offer two examples to demonstrate the point.

I tried a case involving claims of improper care by two orthopedic surgeons of a patient who had developed compartment syndrome of an upper extremity fractured during a work-related accident. I represented the primary surgeon. The assistant surgeon was represented by separate counsel. My

expert was a first-timer. In fact, after defending him in a malpractice action years earlier when he was a young physician
and recommending that after a few more years of practice he
consider serving as an expert, he decided to accept my advice.
Fortunately for me and my client, his testimony was flawless
and his ability to withstand fierce examination by an experienced and highly competent plaintiff's attorney was remarkable. In contrast, the testimony of the co-defendant orthopedic
surgeon's expert was less than compelling. Although I knew
him to be a seasoned trial witness, his demeanor was unexpectedly odd. Before answering numerous questions, including those posed by the attorney who retained him, the witness
would raise his eyes and look at the ceiling as if to gain
divine inspiration. He did this with astounding regularity—so
much so that his entire presentation was damaged. Instead of
appearing confident, he was weak and ineffectual.

In another case, contrary to my pre-testimony instructions, my retained expert felt compelled to repeatedly glance
at me seated at counsel table during cross-examination by
the adverse attorney. He appeared tentative and in need of
reassurance and support. Although his direct testimony was
adequate, his demeanor during my adversary's questioning
revealed a lack of confidence. The effect of his direct testimony was eroded and not by anything he said.

A defense expert who offers damaging testimony in
response to cross-examination may be rehabilitated during
limited redirect examination by retaining counsel. However,
an expert who stares at the ceiling or seeks reassurance from
retaining counsel cannot be told during the course of his or
her testimony to stop doing so. Thus, the damage caused by a
faltering demeanor may not be readily cured.

Finally, expert testimony is delivered from the witness stand
in a seated position. To those who are used to speaking in
more open forums, the restraints imposed by the confines
of the courtroom may prove uncomfortable or unsettling.
I have seen an expert repeatedly tilt his chair back on its
rear legs (tempting fate in the process), and I have witnessed

an expert unknowingly rock his body back and forth in his seat. Both appeared uneasy, and their behavior, at the least, detracted from their testimony. Avoid behavior which is distracting to the jury or may appear to manifest anxiety.

If you believe that portions of your testimony will be more effective if you stand, discuss with retaining counsel how this can be accomplished. You can only do so with the judge's permission and only for good reason. If your testimony requires the use of trial exhibits, the court likely will allow you to stand in front of the jury box. As previously discussed, enlargements of patient records, anatomical drawings, models and computer-based presentations are often used at trial. Their use in conjunction with your testimony can serve as a valid reason for you to leave the witness stand. The result may well be a less staid presentation and a more relaxed performance.

No matter the location from which you testify, always remember to connect with each juror on an individual basis. This topic has already been addressed in significant detail. It bears repeating, however, that you should consider your audience and given its rather small size, speak to and look into the eyes of each jury member at least once during the course of your testimony. Forge an alliance with the jurors on a person-to-person basis and look for a physical reaction from each individual with whom you have connected. A subtle smile or head nod may be an encouraging sign.

Testimony

The malpractice case itself obviously will dictate the substance of your trial testimony. Fashioned by the nature of the plaintiff's claims, your role as an expert was defined at the time of your retention. You may have given expression to that role by crafting an expert report and perhaps by testifying at a deposition. The journey that began at the time you first reviewed file materials will commonly conclude with your trial appearance.

This of course assumes that your opinions have some basis in the science of your practice discipline. If not, adverse counsel may request a formal hearing before a judge to explore the issue by asking you questions about your opinions and their foundation. Here is where the concept of evidence-based medicine has real application. The expert's opinions must be an expression of and based upon recognized scientific principles. Opinions which reflect only the individual thinking of an expert without foundation in the science of that expert's profession should not and will not be permitted. A successful challenge to an expert's opinions based upon the lack of a true recognized scientific foundation for those opinions will prevent that expert from ever testifying at trial.

Absent such a challenge, offering your opinions at trial first requires that the trial judge qualify you as an expert in your field. Consequently, direct examination will begin with questions about your professional credentials. Although qualification as an expert may vary slightly from jurisdiction to jurisdiction, at a minimum, you will have to testify about your education, training and professional experience. Opposing counsel then will be given an opportunity to conduct limited *"voir dire"*, that is, elicit testimony about your background in an effort to establish that you lack the requisite credentials to be considered an expert or that you possess only minimal credentials. That said, however, rarely will an expert be precluded from testifying. It is for this reason that some attorneys disfavor conducting *voir dire* and will wait until substantive cross-examination to ask credential-related questions.

If *voir dire* does elicit testimony that permits a legitimate challenge to the witness's qualifications as an expert, something has gone terribly awry. (Perhaps the retaining lawyer hired the wrong expert or the expert somehow miscommunicated his credentials at the time he was retained, either of which should have been detected long before trial.) The liability expert is the lynchpin of a malpractice trial, and if the court refuses to permit an expert to testify, the defense may be irreparably damaged. Even if other experts are available, an attorney never wants to present a witness to the jury only to have the judge reject the witness as unqualified. The negative psychological effect of such a development is not easily overcome.

Voir dire, however, can serve to impair an expert's impact by revealing weaknesses in the expert's credentials such as the absence of (1) professional honors or awards; (2) hospital departmental or committee positions; (3) academic appointments or (4) relevant publications and presentations. As further examples, you could be confronted with the following facts: (1) you were denied admission to American medical schools; (2) you never participated in a relevant residency and/or fellowship program; (3) your hospital privileges were temporarily suspended or (4) you only devote a small portion of your professional time to seeing patients clinically. Of course, questions of this type should be anticipated, and all potential weaknesses in your presentation should be discussed with the retaining lawyer before the day you take the stand. Then, plans can be fashioned to minimize the effect of such negative testimony. Those plans might include neutralizing the effect of such testimony by first disclosing the troublesome issues during direct examination. Let me use two examples to prove the point.

If retaining counsel elicits testimony about the suspension of hospital privileges rather than the adverse attorney, it may sound like this:

Question: How long have you been affiliated with ABC Medical Center?
Answer: Ten years.

Question: What type of privileges do you have?
Answer: Full attending privileges.

Question: Have you had those privileges on an uninterrupted basis throughout?
Answer: No.

Question: Why not?

Answer: Seven years ago, my partner became rather ill and for about a month, I was taking care of both his patients and my patients. Because I was so busy, I didn't have a chance to sign the hospital discharge summaries for some of our practice's hospital patients as quickly as the hospital required, and so my privileges were temporarily suspended for a period of 24 hours. Once I signed the discharge summaries, my privileges were restored.

A second example might be handled this way if retaining counsel addresses the issue first:

Question: Do you devote all your professional time to the clinical practice of medicine?

Answer: No. I spend only some of my time seeing patients in the office.

Question: Why is that?

Answer: I am an Associate Professor at XYZ University Medical School and spend roughly 40% of my professional time teaching. For the past six years, I also have given lectures nationally, and approximately 20% of my time is spent as an invited guest lecturer at medical schools throughout the country.

Much better, right?

Once the court accepts the liability expert, the retaining attorney will resume his direct examination. Typically, after confirming retention by the questioning lawyer to review the matter as an expert, the witness will itemize the materials examined and indicate that he formulated opinions based on that review. Retaining counsel will then pose questions designed to explore the relevant facts and issues and to elicit related opinions. (Such is the case whether the witness is a plaintiff or defense expert.) Remember that your direct testimony should not look rehearsed, even though you and retaining counsel should have carefully prepared before-hand. Instead, your presentation should resemble a dialog and appear somewhat spontaneous to the jury. Your answers should appear genuine and not staged.

If you have written a report and you have it with you, you may be tempted to refer to it, worse yet, actually read directly from it during your direct testimony. Avoid the temptation. First, this makes you look less confident. In many jurisdictions, you will not be permitted to just read passages from your report. You should know the contents of your report, and you should know your own opinions. If you need to review the report to refresh your memory, that exercise should be completed before you step foot in the courtroom.

The liability expert ultimately will identify the standard of care that governed the defendant's conduct at the time treatment was rendered and will state that the defendant comported with that standard of care. As a natural consequence of such testimony, often the defense expert will also comment on causation, that is, state that the defendant's conduct did not cause or contribute to the claimed injuries. If, however, the expert is not qualified or not competent to address causation, another expert retained for such purpose will address the issue.

Although it is difficult to predict how other defense attorneys will approach the examination of the factual issues with their experts, it makes sense to expect that it will follow some reasonable chronological order. Of course, as discussed, having participated in a pre-testimony meeting, you should know how counsel plans to conduct direct examination. Generally, it is a fair bet that all relevant opinions expressed to the retaining lawyer will be the subject of testimony. If you read key imaging studies as part of your assignment, expect to show them to the jury and testify about your interpretation. If an Independent Medical Examination (IME) was conducted, a portion of the presentation will focus on the performance of the IME, your findings and their impact on your opinions.

The length of the direct examination will be governed by a number of factors, including, but not necessarily limited to: (1) the factual context of the criticized care; (2) the number of defendants on whose behalf you have been retained; (3) the number of issues reviewed; (4) the complexity of the issues; (5) the volume of material reviewed and (6) the number and complexity of opinions to be offered. It may last 60 minutes or three hours.

After direct examination is concluded, adverse counsel will conduct cross-examination. Cross-examination can be as short as ten minutes (I've seen it) or as long as five hours (I've done it). Expect cross to be generally related to your direct testimony and rather pointed. You also may be asked about opinions that might naturally flow from those offered during direct testimony but which you may have deliberately avoided because of their potentially harmful impact on the defendant for whom you are testifying. Further, adverse counsel typically is entitled to explore opinions contained in your report or offered at deposition, even if they were not expressly stated during direct testimony.

Counsel may also inquire about opinions offered by you as an expert in other matters involving similar issues where the opinions might be inconsistent with those now advanced. Of course, such questions typically are prompted by adverse counsel's prior investigation of reports or depositions from other cases available to the plaintiff's bar. Suffice it to say, if such opinions exist, this is not the moment when retaining counsel should first hear them. As mentioned earlier, full disclosure of inconsistent opinions is essential at the time of initial contact or as soon thereafter as is possible. This is a continuing obligation assumed by the expert, and any lapse can be devastating if the inconsistency is used by adverse counsel at trial. Having once been in that position, I can assure you that hearing at trial (for the first time) a retained expert confirm a contrary opinion offered in an earlier matter is stunning.

Substantive cross-examination will differ from trial to trial, as a result of each matter's unique fact pattern. However, some common themes are worth mentioning. To the extent that your opinions are based on the underlying facts, the use of slightly skewed or incomplete facts during direct testimony will be highlighted during cross-examination. Opinions based on the acceptance of the defendant's version of events as opposed to the plaintiff's version may be explored and exposed. The absence of adequate documentation by the defendant about significant events may be pursued. As well, adverse counsel may ask you to acknowledge as at least a possibility that which you believe to be improbable. In fact, the more frequently you concede as at least possible that which the plaintiff's expert has testified as probable, the better for the plaintiff.

Also, expect the occasional use of the "hypothetical question", that is, a question which incorporates a series of facts favorable to the plaintiff, after which a conclusory statement is recited with which you are asked to agree. Typically, disagreement is difficult, because adverse counsel cleverly uses only the facts that naturally and logically prompt the stated conclusion. Of course, if you are truly unable to agree given the deliberately confining nature of the question, say so. However, you cannot refuse to answer a hypothetical question simply because the adverse lawyer has utilized only "plaintiff-friendly" facts or omitted a fact you consider critical. Respond to the question and if your answer is damaging to the defense, expect retaining counsel to revisit the issue during redirect examination.

An important difference between direct and cross-examination is that on cross-examination, an opposing lawyer may use "leading questions", whereas on direct, retaining counsel may not. Questions asked during direct examination must not point to an answer. On cross, they may, and the attorney will attempt to "lead" the witness to that answer. Thus, a "leading question" is one in which the questioning attorney does the "testifying" and the fact sought to be established is contained in the question itself requiring only a yes or no response. For example, a question posed by defense counsel of a plaintiff's expert might sound like this: "The plaintiff failed to provide a complete medical history to the defendant during the first office visit, isn't that so?" Cross-examination routinely incorporates leading questions, and an effective cross relies heavily on the leading question to control the witness.

Of course, if a question cannot be legitimately answered with a yes or no response, say so. Don't permit adverse counsel to box you in with a prefatory instruction that you respond yes or no to a given question. If a reasoned and intelligent answer precludes a simple yes or no, it is unlikely that the trial judge will force you to provide the one-word response questioning counsel seeks.

Understand that the tenor of the cross will be dictated by the personality of the questioning attorney. Lawyers have different styles, and during your expert career, you will learn how to best handle each variation. No matter the approach, however, a plaintiff's attorney knows the importance of the liability defense expert. Accordingly, expect a vigorous cross-examination.

The manner in which you respond to cross-examination and the cross-examiner will be determined, in part, by your personality and what you have learned over time works best with the jury. Never lose sight of the fact that the battle between you and opposing counsel, no matter how heated, is on display. The jury can see everything. Don't let adverse counsel "push your buttons". Always maintain your composure. Avoid being abrasive or smug. Don't be flip or glib and never be disrespectful or impatient. In a difficult spot during cross-examination, rely on who you are and what you know. Attorneys become attorneys by graduating from law school and passing a bar exam. That's it. With rare exception, lawyers, even those who specialize in malpractice, don't have the education, training and experience possessed by you. They can't know what you know and therefore can't go "toe to toe" with you. During tough cross, fall back on what made you an expert in your field and use it.

Proper courtroom conduct after your testimony is completed deserves comment. My remarks in this regard are prompted by having witnessed, from time to time, utterly inappropriate behavior by plaintiffs' experts after testimony is completed.

When you finish testifying, gather your materials from the witness stand. Leave behind all trial exhibits used during your testimony. As you step down from the witness stand, do not speak to the jury. Don't thank them. Don't say goodbye. Don't say have a nice day. Don't say anything. You may, of course, smile slightly, but that's it. As you pass counsel table, say nothing to the attorneys and do not stop to whisper to the lawyer who retained you or to return materials he supplied.

Return to your seat in the courtroom. Do not head directly for the exit door. Running out of the courtroom as soon as you step down from the witness stand gives the impression that you just can't wait to get out of there. It may also support the unsavory notion that you may just be a "witness for hire". You do not want the jury to believe that since your testimony is over and your billing meter has stopped, you need to bolt.

Most likely, the judge will recess briefly after your testimony and permit the jury to relax for a few minutes. If that should happen, wait for the jury to leave the courtroom before you do or say anything. Once every juror has departed, you may then approach the attorney who retained you or simply leave. If the court does not take a recess after your testimony, but instead directs counsel to call the next witness, wait a few minutes and then quietly leave without spectacle.

Let me explain what prompts these recommendations.

As a trial witness, your role is to answer questions. If you're not being asked a question, it's improper for you to speak. It's even worse when your unsolicited remarks, no matter how well-intentioned or polite, are directed toward the jury when your service as a witness is over.

Verbal communication with retaining counsel is equally egregious. The jury should only see your exchange with counsel when you are testifying. Jurors should not speculate as to your hushed remarks as you leave. The impression may contradict the idea that you are objective and intellectually independent. Do you want the jury to think you're saying, "How'd I do?" or "Mail me the check." I can't imagine anything so important that it has to be said at that moment. Neither will the jury. At the very least, your need to chat with counsel as you depart will be received by the jury as "odd" and incongruous. That is not the impression you want to leave.

There also is no reason to deposit materials on counsel table as you walk by. That too will be seen as strange and will invite speculation by the jurors as to what's in the materials or why the expert left them with counsel. Again, it's likely to undercut the image that you are independent, which is central to your credibility. Either take the documents with you or, if it's urgent, wait for a recess to return the materials.

I stated at the outset that courtroom demeanor is critical. Don't spoil effective testimony with lapses in your demeanor as you leave.

It also bears mentioning that people outside the courtroom with whom you have fleeting contact when you appear for trial could be jurors. This may occur as you enter or exit the courthouse, the elevator, the restroom, the building cafeteria or the neighborhood restaurant. You should refrain from making statements about the case in which you're participating, no matter how innocuous, because a juror may overhear them. Nor should you be seen hobnobbing with attorneys during breaks including those with whom you may be acquainted.

At some point after you testify (typically after the trial's conclusion), you will likely be contacted by defense counsel concerning the outcome of the trial. Use that occasion to obtain feedback about your testimony. If succeeding as an expert is important to you, the insight gained by speaking to counsel will be invaluable. Regardless of whether the defendant won or lost, ask the attorney to spend a few minutes critiquing you. Learn from your experience. Correct what needs to be improved and apply what worked to your next court appearance.

Finally, do not discard or delete your file until you have confirmed with defense counsel that you may do so. After trial, a motion for a new trial and/or an appeal may be filed by one of the parties. If the case has to be tried again, expect to appear as a witness at the new proceeding.

Chapter 8

Creating an Effective Curriculum Vitae

Without question, your Curriculum Vitae (CV) is critical to a successful expert career. It will define you, and its contents must fairly reflect who you are professionally. It will open doors and get you noticed. Further, as a recitation of credentials, it will be used to enhance your credibility as a witness. The CV serves to identify a practitioner as an expert in a given field and should provide a basis upon which to present opinions. Ultimately, jurors scrutinize an expert's credentials in determining the weight to give that expert's opinions. With so much riding on the CV, it behooves you to make it as effective as possible. Do not, however, exaggerate.

Importantly, a CV is not a resume. The latter typically is used to support an application for a job, position or privileges and, therefore, routinely contains personal information, self-serving comments about special skills and descriptions of certain professional experiences, none of which should be recited in a CV.

In addition to listing your name, professional mailing and email addresses and practice specialty, the CV should contain the following information.

Education and Training

List the names and locations of all schools attended after high school. Unless your high school was regionally or nationally notorious, its inclusion is unnecessary. Indicate the years of attendance at or years of graduation from undergraduate, graduate and medical schools. Identify special education programs you attended and significant scholastic honors and awards you received. Internships, residencies and fellowships should be mentioned. Include the nature, years and locations of your training. Again, if you received special recognition, honors or awards during your training, your CV should recite them.

Board Certification

Board certification is key. List the name of the specialty board, the year of certification and the year(s) of re-certification, if applicable. I don't typically recommend listing board eligibility only because it serves to highlight the fact that you are not board certified.

Hospital Affiliations

Identify all hospitals with which you currently are affiliated. List hospital names and locales, the nature of your privileges, if other than full attending and years of affiliation. Institutions with which you were associated in the past can be included if the termination of your privileges did not result from adverse action taken by the hospital. For example, if you moved your practice or voluntarily decided to limit the number of hospitals where you work for your convenience or to enhance patient care, identifying hospitals (with years of affiliation) where you no longer have privileges is acceptable.

Particularly important positions held at hospitals also should be included in your CV. Department or division chair, chief or director posts with years of service should be listed. So should significant hospital committee memberships or offices (with years of service).

Academic Positions

Although a pure academician who does not have clinical experience rarely serves as an expert in a routine malpractice action, a practicing clinician who has taught or who teaches is attractive to attorneys and jurors alike. Consequently, if your background includes academic experience, list it. Identify the institution by name and location, your position and years of service.

Professional Organizations

Include all professional organizations, associations and societies with which you are affiliated. Membership in defunct organizations or those to which you no longer belong typically should not be listed. If you hold or have held an important position in an organization, identify it and the years of service.

Military Experience

If you have served or currently serve in a branch of the military, National Guard or Reserves, absolutely include this information. As a general statement, jurors respect the military, and, as one who has served or continues to serve, you will likely gain immediate respect by the jury. If you have served in a war theater or have seen military action, your stature will be further enhanced. If you have provided medical care during a war, this fact also should be reflected in your CV. Include significant decorations received from the military, as well.

Awards and Honors

Professional citations of almost any type are worth mentioning in your CV. List the nature of the award or honor, the name of the entity that bestowed it and the date of receipt. If a short description of the accolade would help a layperson understand its significance, include it.

Publications, Presentations, Seminars and Lectures

Especially attractive are works that you have published, presentations to other practitioners, and seminars and lectures given on professional topics. Listed publications should include books, book chapters, articles and abstracts. Full titles of the publications and publication years should be included. Presentations, seminars and lectures similarly should be completely described and should include dates.

Athletic Program Affiliations

If you have held or hold a position with an athletic program or sports franchise, you are wise to identify it.

For example, an association with a professional, semi-professional, college or even high school sports team is invaluable. If you are the podiatrist for a soccer team, the orthopedist for a football team or the chiropractor for a gymnastics team, you may be accorded instant credibility by those who support the team or the sport and perhaps by those who don't. After all, you must truly be an expert in feet and ankles, if you are the podiatrist for an entire soccer team. So the thinking goes.

Public Service

By its very designation, this type of credential is defined by jurors in a most positive way. Therefore, if you have served the public in some fashion, your CV should reflect it. For example, if you participate in school-sponsored programs, mention it. If you have participated in the local police department's D.A.R.E. (Drug Abuse Resistance Education) program by teaching children about the impact drugs have on the body, include it. An ophthalmologist who conducts free annual eye exams provides a valuable public service. Again, your public-mindedness will be well received by jurors and will tend to enhance the impression that you are "high-minded" and therefore reliable.

Media Appearances

Invited guest appearances on television, radio programs or podcasts are also worth including in your CV. If you hosted such programs, all the better. Like service to a sports team, your participation in such programming suggests that you have been selected because you are particularly capable. Such appearances will promote the perception that you are a distinguished member of your profession. They further reveal that you are good or, at least, experienced at public speaking and are eloquent or charismatic. It makes sense to surmise that producers have hired you for these qualities.

Chapter 9

Getting Started

Realize that the defense bar will not necessarily know who you are or that you have an interest in serving as a malpractice defense expert. The onus, therefore, is on you to convey that interest and "market" yourself. Although there may be occasions when an attorney you know will ask if you're interested in malpractice expert work, the likelihood that this will happen is remote. Certainly, you should not rely on such a happenstance occurrence if indeed you are serious. Be aggressive. Embark on a marketing campaign that will bring your name and credentials to the attention of members of the defense bar.

Suggested below are various approaches to this effort. Try some or all of them. Some methods are expense-free. The simplest and most economic approach is verbal communication. Speaking to people who can help you obtain malpractice expert work requires little effort and virtually no expense. The individuals whom you might approach are varied and all should be considered. Other methods, such as advertisements, mass mailings and websites, will require the expenditure of funds.

Frankly, it doesn't matter which method you first employ. You may sequence your marketing plan or you may choose to use multiple methods simultaneously. The decision as to how and in what order to proceed is purely personal. Do what is comfortable and affordable. Remember, all you need is that first case. If you do well, your reputation will grow, as will your work.

Your Malpractice Attorney

If you have been in the unwelcome position of being a defendant in a malpractice case, you already know an attorney who can be of great assistance to you. If that lawyer's practice is significantly devoted to handling malpractice cases, he or she will have an ongoing need for malpractice experts. Further, the attorney may know other malpractice defense lawyers and, more important, people associated with the malpractice insurance carriers from which defense assignments are received. The fact that you were a defendant in a malpractice case (or in multiple cases) will not in and of itself cause counsel to shy away from retaining you as an expert. It is a fact of modern-day professional life that even top notch practitioners are sued. Simply having been a defendant will not prevent you from becoming a valued expert.

Understand that the response you get from counsel to your inquiry will be greatly affected by your CV and how well you responded to examination at deposition and/or at trial by adverse counsel in your case. If your performance was compelling or you were perceived as having expert potential, you likely will be supported in this endeavor.

Though infrequent, there are times when a malpractice defendant is so impressive as a trial witness that he carries the day himself. The trial is won on the sheer ability of the defendant to "wow" the jury. It is unusual that the defendant is a better witness than the retained liability expert, but it happens. I was involved in an orthopedic malpractice case that resulted in my representing a young orthopedic surgeon whose credentials were only surpassed by his good looks, charm and communication skills. (I alluded to him earlier.) In aid of my client's defense, I retained the services of an experienced, knowledgeable and trial-capable liability expert in the field of orthopedics. As well as he did in court, the defense verdict was as much due to the testimony of the defendant as it was that of the expert. The defendant impressed the jury with his credentials, his knowledge of the "medicine", his ability to communicate and his capacity to respond quickly and convincingly to tough cross-examination.

When the case ended, I inquired of my client as to his interest in serving as a malpractice expert for me in the future. He was agreeable. His youth prevented me from using his services immediately. However, within three years of that experience, I retained him for his first case and recommended him to the representatives of the malpractice insurance carriers with whom I did business. In fact, he was so capable in his first court appearance as an expert for me that an attorney representing a co-defendant promptly retained him to serve as a defense expert in another matter he was handling. Over time, this practitioner developed into an effective and accomplished witness with a reputation as a top-level expert.

On another occasion, I represented an obstetrician in defense of a case in which it was alleged that he had improperly delayed a baby's delivery causing brain damage. This physician was an established member of his profession who had significant accomplishments to his credit and who had recently relinquished his private practice to become affiliated with a regional medical center in an administrative capacity. Although he also had been a defendant in prior malpractice matters, this was my first encounter with him. I had no direct knowledge of his ability as a trial witness. I only knew that he made a strong personal appearance, was amiable and bright.

During the trial, which was emotionally charged given the subject matter, effective cross-examination of various expert witnesses for the plaintiffs had somewhat crippled their case, forcing the plaintiffs' attorney to make an unexpected move. As the morning session opened on the fourth day of trial, everyone had anticipated that another of the plaintiffs' experts would be the opening witness. Although my client was prepared to testify, it was expected that he would testify as my initial witness, rather than as a witness during the plaintiffs' case-in-chief. However, the plaintiffs' attorney called my client to the stand as his first witness of the day. Evidently, in an effort to catch my client off guard and recapture the momentum of the trial, the plaintiffs' attorney called him unexpectedly and attempted to discredit him. The plaintiffs' lawyer was unsuccessful. My client seized the moment and controlled the examination and the examiner. In fact, the plaintiffs' attorney's gamble failed miserably. The defendant was anything but rattled by the surprise attack. Instead, given an early opportunity to testify, my client clearly described the subject events and calmly explained his reasoning for decisions made. Ultimately, we enjoyed a defense verdict.

In light of his performance, I subsequently retained my former client as a defense expert in another matter and recommended him to my insurance carrier clients. Over the years, he has repeatedly served as an expert both for me and other malpractice attorneys.

These are but two examples of where a defendant in a malpractice case has turned an unpleasant lawsuit experience into a positive opportunity. You can do the same. Even if your lawyer doesn't approach you about serving as a malpractice expert, that doesn't mean you're incapable of doing so or that he won't support you. Initiate conversation about it and express your interest. Ask your attorney to inform other malpractice defense lawyers of your availability. More important, ask him to communicate your interest and transmit your CV to the insurance carrier representatives with whom he deals. A positive endorsement from an attorney who routinely interacts with malpractice insurance companies will be of immense help in developing expert work.

Liability Carriers/Brokers

Akin to speaking to your malpractice attorney is communicating directly with your malpractice carrier and/or broker. These contacts can be a valuable source of expert work. If you have been a defendant in a malpractice matter, it's likely that you have already interacted with a representative of your liability insurance carrier. If so, a telephone call advising of your interest in doing malpractice work is a good first step. Follow up with a confirming email or letter transmitting a copy of your CV. Invite the representative to contact your attorney, or, better yet, also call the attorney and ask that he communicate directly with the representative about how well you performed in your lawsuit.

I also recommend contacting professional liability carriers other than your own. Communicate with companies that provided coverage in the past, those that you have learned of while attempting to secure coverage and those that have solicited your insurance business. To obtain a complete list of insurance carriers authorized to conduct business in a state of interest, google that state's insurance department. To secure a more tailored list, contact the state's medical, podiatric or chiropractic societies. National, state and local specialty organizations should also be contacted, as they likely can provide carrier information as well. Once you have identified the carriers you intend to pursue, email each company's Vice President of Claims or Claims Manager and/or transmit an email or letter of introduction with a CV.

There have been occasions when the carriers with which I have worked have emailed me about a practitioner interested in serving as a malpractice expert. That email usually has an attached copy of the practitioner's CV and an endorsement from the carrier. When you contact a carrier, you should ask how to secure such an endorsement.

Another way to gain exposure to the defense bar and malpractice carriers is to provide "peer review" services as a consultant—rather than a testifying expert—in connection with malpractice lawsuits. Some carriers have a peer review program that involves practitioners in virtually every specialty. The purpose typically is to secure an expert opinion about the merits of a given case early in the litigation. Some carriers involve the defendant, defense counsel and a carrier representative in the review process by convening a meeting where a frank discussion about the criticized care occurs. Typically, the reviewing practitioner examines the relevant treatment records, poses questions to the defendant about the issues raised by the litigation and offers opinions about liability, causation and/or damages.

Other carriers use a less involved process, preferring simply to furnish the relevant treatment records to a specialty practitioner for review and written assessment. The resulting analysis will address liability, causation and/or damages issues and provide guidance as to potential defenses and the advisability of other specialty reviews. It may also make recommendations as to treatment records and other documents that should be secured during discovery.

Regardless of the intricacies of the process, the point is, the program only works with the participation of willing practitioners who can take the time needed to make the process meaningful. Review practitioners provide a valuable and much-appreciated service, and like litigation work itself, it is professionally gratifying. Of course, there usually is a financial incentive as well, such as an hourly fee, or an insurance premium credit or rate discount if the insurance company is your malpractice carrier.

Acting as a reviewer will preclude your participation as an expert in any case reviewed by you, and it may even prevent you from serving as an expert in any matter involving that carrier. Some carriers prefer that practitioners who serve as reviewers refrain from acting as litigation experts. This approach insulates the review process from discovery and promotes the confidential disclosure of opinions about the substantive allegations by the review practitioner. Nevertheless, providing this service can open doors. Impressing the carrier's representative, defense counsel and/ or the defendant is a sure first step to developing a positive reputation in the defense arena. The more frequently you serve in this capacity, the greater the likelihood that you will be considered as a potential defense expert in other matters. If you are able to demonstrate a facility as a reviewing practitioner, your name will circulate among insurance carrier representatives and defense attorneys, and expert assignments will follow.

Another approach to securing expert work may be to contact your insurance broker. If your broker has a reasonably good relationship with your malpractice carrier (and other carriers), enlisting the broker's help may be valuable. Brokers in this field may have a long and solid history with their carriers and typically enjoy personal relationships with carrier staff. At a minimum, a broker should be able to provide the names and addresses of carriers you can approach.

Colleagues, Patients and Attorneys

Fellow practitioners, patients and attorneys with whom you are acquainted may all serve as fertile marketing targets, even if only informally. As mentioned, the power of word of mouth cannot be overstated. Nor can the strength of those relationships that you currently enjoy.

Professional colleagues certainly should be approached, especially those who do expert work. Indeed, you may know practitioners who serve or have served as malpractice experts. Let them know of your interest and availability and ask for the names of attorneys or insurance carrier contacts. Better yet, if you are sufficiently friendly with the colleague, ask that he approach the people with whom he has worked to provide an endorsement. Furnish copies of your CV for transmittal to such individuals. Of course, follow up such effort with both an introductory email and/or telephone call.

Quite fortuitously, patients in your practice may be attorneys or individuals in the insurance business. Learn more about them during the course of office encounters. You may find that they are involved in the malpractice field or know people who are. Advise them of your interest in serving as a malpractice expert and explore their professional malpractice needs or the relationships they have which may prove advantageous to you. Always have copies of your CV available in your office and offer one to your patient. Of course, follow-up is important. Initiate contact a few days later and ask what more you can do in furtherance of your interest.

In addition to attorneys who are your patients, you may be familiar with other attorneys who you might approach. Whether they are friends, friends of friends or your own lawyers in matters unrelated to malpractice, they should be contacted. Chances are they know of malpractice defense attorneys whom they can call on your behalf. Again, provide a copy of your CV and follow up on all leads identified by such attorneys.

Advertisement

An additional component of your marketing plan may be advertising. This tool may be highly effective and should be seriously considered. Attorneys in need of an expert in a given matter may consult advertisements, and, given the plethora of expert ads in legal publications, one can surmise that they work. Be aware, however, that plaintiffs' attorneys, more frequently than defense counsel, consult such advertisements. Further, it is not inexpensive. Therefore, I recommend that you contact individuals who have placed such ads and inquire of their success before doing so yourself.

Typically, ads of this type are placed in legal publications that target lawyers. They may appear in specially designated sections that carry ads by various types of experts available to serve in litigated matters or they may be randomly but conspicuously placed elsewhere in the publication. Ad size and type will dictate the cost.

Various professional publications are available. Check with the bar association of the states in which you want to serve to obtain a list of the publications directed to attorneys. At a minimum, you should consider advertising in the legal newspaper(s) covering legal news in a given state. Typically, this publication is weekly and likely enjoys the largest subscription numbers. In New Jersey, for example, the weekly legal newspaper is the *New Jersey Law Journal.* It behooves you to investigate subscription numbers of the weekly newspapers of interest.

Annually, *The National Law Journal* publishes an online national directory of medical experts as well as online directories of expert witnesses for various geographic regions, including New Jersey, Mid-Atlantic, Midwestern, New England, New York, Southeastern, Southwestern and Western. These directories identify experts by specialty in nearly every discipline and serve as a reference source for attorneys seeking expert assistance. Additionally, the directories contain full-page Curricula Vitae and several display ads of various experts. While you must pay a fee to be listed, having your name in this publication may be advantageous. The website www.almexperts.com is where attorneys can locate experts by specialty. Your listing can link the browser to your CV, a profile, a photograph, your individual website and your email address. Appearing in the website, therefore, may prove an excellent marketing tool.

Similar information can be posted in the JurisPro Expert Witness Directory (www.jurispro.com), a free online directory of experts in almost any field. This website allows browsers to obtain detailed information about listed experts, including linked individual websites. Photographs of experts are typically posted and streaming audio allows visitors to hear the expert speak.

The New Jersey Lawyers Diary, which is a reference guide used by lawyers in New Jersey, also publishes *The Legal Pages* annually. This book contains expert listings and advertisements and is worth investigating. *The Legal Pages* also offers a website, www.lawdiary.com, on which ads can be placed.

Every jurisdiction has legal specialty organizations that publish magazines, newspapers and/or newsletters, all of which likely welcome advertisers. Typically, the personal injury bar and the defense bar in a given state have separate organizations that promote their interests and those of the clients they represent. You can learn about them by contacting state bar associations. Again, investigate subscription numbers before purchasing ad space.

Finally, state bar associations usually publish a monthly or quarterly magazine. Here too, advertisements abound. Although you might consider placing an ad in such a magazine, it is probably less likely that an attorney in need of a malpractice expert will consult such a magazine than a current edition of his or her jurisdiction's weekly legal newspaper.

Importantly, if you advertise your services, be prepared to be questioned about it at deposition and/or at trial. Whether your participation in a given matter is the result of an ad or not, the fact that you market yourself in this fashion will be exploited by adverse counsel. By eliciting testimony about the publications in which you advertise, the length of time you have advertised and the states in which you advertise, the opposing lawyer will try to establish that you are nothing more than an opportunist who will say what needs to be said for a price. A "true" expert, adverse counsel will suggest, is one who somehow is discovered by the retaining attorney based on reputation and not because of a highly visible newspaper ad.

I must say that, having used this tactic myself, it can be quite effective in discrediting an opposing expert. The greater the number of ads in a given publication, the greater the number of publications used by the expert, the greater the number of jurisdictions in which the expert advertises and the greater the number of years ads have been used, the greater the likelihood that adverse examination about such matters will prove effective.

As a result, advertisements create an inherent dilemma. On the one hand, they may garner work. On the other hand, they may negatively affect an expert's credibility. Deciding what to do requires assessing individual circumstances. If you are just getting started and have either opted against other marketing methods or have enjoyed little success with them, advertising might be explored. Many practitioners begin their expert careers using ads and, after developing work, stop using them. Some practitioners use ads to "jump start" a stalled expert career and then end their use after their expert career is renewed. Others rely heavily on advertisements long term for the development and growth of business. Such practitioners and the attorneys who retain them care little about the inevitable examination by adverse counsel about their advertising efforts either because it is believed that the collateral damage is minimal and/or that the other qualities the expert "brings to the table" outweigh the negative impact of such examination.

Expert Agencies

Organizations established to assist attorneys in finding experts exist in almost every state, and some cross state lines. Some of these entities provide the names and credentials of experts for review by lawyers. Others offer a full array of services, including matching the malpractice case to the appropriate expert from an internal database of available practitioners, supplying the attorney with that expert's CV, reviewing and summarizing medical records, forwarding materials to the expert and securing a report from the expert for the attorney. Expert agencies typically charge the retaining attorney a fee for these services. However, there may be a fee charged to the expert for listing his or her name and making it available to malpractice lawyers.

Such services often print ads in the publications mentioned above in the same way individual practitioners do. Such entities may email ads and brochures to lawyers engaged in personal injury practice generally or specializing in malpractice litigation specifically. Frequently, they have rather informative websites designed to attract attorneys in need of experts.

Like direct advertising, such agency listings will likely be the subject of effective examination by adverse counsel at deposition and/or trial. As a result, the potential for collateral damage exists, especially for practitioners who are listed with or who have obtained assignments from multiple agencies in multiple jurisdictions for a number of years. However, as with direct advertisements, proceeding with this method requires the practitioner to balance the benefits against the potential detriment.

Assuming you decide to become listed, you can locate the service or services with which to become affiliated by reviewing the expert portion of the classified section of the weekly (or monthly) legal newspapers in the states of interest. There, you likely will find the names of various organizations offering their services to attorneys. Specialty legal publications—which you can identify through state bar associations—also will have such listings. Without even obtaining a copy of the publication of interest, you may be able to contact the offices of the publication and request the names of the expert organizations that place ads. In the alternative, you can contact your attorney or perhaps an attorney who has represented you in a malpractice case and ask for the names of prominent agencies.

Some of the referral agencies that might help you get started include:

1. American Medical Experts (www.americanmedicalexperts. com or 888-678-3973) Aldie, VA;
2. American Medical Forensic Specialists, Inc. (AMFS) (www.amfs.com or 800-275-8903) Walnut Creek, CA;
3. Consolidated Consultants Co. (www.freereferral.com or 800-683-9847) Chula Vista, CA;
4. Expert Institute (www.expertinstitute.com or 888-858-9511) New York, NY;
5. ExpertPages (www.expertpages.com or 800-380-8898) Sausalito, CA;
6. Forensic Group, Inc. (www.forensicgroup.com or 800-555-5422) Pasadena, CA;
7. IMS Expert Services (www.ims-expertservices.com or 877-838-8464) Pensacola, FL;
8. JD MD Inc. (www.jdmd.com or 800-225-5363) Jackson, MS;
9. Medical Advisors, Inc. (www.techmedexperts.com or 800-666-7045) Blue Bell, PA;
10. Medilex, Inc. (www.medilexinc.com or 212-234-1999) New York, NY;
11. Med League Support Services Inc. (www.medleague.com or 908-788-8227) Flemington, NJ;
12. MedQuest, Ltd. (www.medquestltd.com or 800-633-6251) New York, NY;
13. Physicians For Quality (www.pfq.com or 800-284-3627) San Marcos, TX;
14. SEAK (www.seak.com or 508-457-1111) Falmouth, MA;
15. TASAmed (www.tasanet.com or 800-523-2319) Blue Bell, PA; and
16. Wendell O. Scott, M.D., LLC Consulting (www.wosmd.com or 908-830-9980) New Providence, NJ.

Mass Mailings

This approach has its appeal in the sheer number of attorneys you can directly contact. With a standard introductory letter or email and CV, you can convey your interest and your credentials at the same time. The problem with this method is that such mass mailings may be discarded or deleted before the attorney really considers their contents. For this reason, you must do something to grab the lawyer's attention. Be unique, be imaginative, get noticed.

A state's *Lawyers Diary*, or equivalent publication, can assist in the creation of a mailing list. Information about such mailing lists can be obtained by visiting www.lawdiary.com.

You can also obtain a list of attorneys by visiting Martindale-Hubbell's www.lawyers.com or www.martindale.com, which will display the names and addresses of attorneys who engage in malpractice litigation in your geographic area of interest. However, Martindale-Hubbell does not list all attorneys in a given practice area. Rather, it lists only those who have paid a fee to be listed. Although you should not rely on Martindale-Hubbell exclusively, it may be a good starting point.

Indeed, there are other organizations that, for a price, will provide mailing lists of attorneys in each state. Depending on where you are looking, there may even be lists based on geographic area or, more important, lists based on practice specialty. Start with the state bar associations. If they don't have the names you need, they may be able to direct you to an entity that does.

Websites

Practitioners typically have websites which provide information about the practice and its members. Attorneys and insurance carriers can make great use of them to learn about experts or prospective experts, especially when they can be linked to expert directory websites of the type mentioned earlier. As a result, a website is an important marketing tool for you. Your website might include information about your interest and availability to serve as an expert in malpractice matters. Posting a photograph certainly is recommended. You also may choose to include streaming audio or streaming video. Again, it is that first case that you seek and the website may be its source.

Reference your website in any communication seeking expert work, including mass mailings. Although your CV, or its equivalent, may be on your website, I recommend that you include or attach a copy with any introductory effort. Don't expect attorneys or insurance representatives to go to your website merely because it's referenced in a communication you send them.

Chapter 10

Rules of Conduct

I hope that having come to this point in the book, you are comfortable with the mechanics of malpractice expert service and understand how to become a valued member of the defense team. If you decide to do expert work, you should be mindful that, as with any professional activity, there are ethical and legal "rules" that circumscribe your conduct.

Over the years, many professional boards and organizations including, but not limited to, the American Society of Anesthesiologists, the American Academy of Neurology, the American Academy of Ophthalmology, the American Academy of Orthopaedic Surgeons, the American Academy of Pediatrics, the American Academy of Physical Medicine and Rehabilitation, the American Association of Neurological Surgeons, the American College of Obstetricians and Gynecologists, the American College of Occupational and Environmental Medicine, the American College of Physicians, the American College of Radiology and the American College of Surgeons have issued policy statements, some more detailed than others, regarding the topic of expert service.

Without question, problems will arise from the failure to adhere to applicable behavioral guidelines. You may damage the legal defense for which you have been retained. You also may expose yourself to investigation by your specialty organization or worse yet, disciplinary action by your state's licensing board.

First and foremost, never accept an assignment where you do not believe you are truly an expert. By that I mean participate in matters only where the specialty at issue is yours and/or your qualifications and experience enable you to make an informed examination and to opine with genuine authority. Often emphasized in the policy statements referenced above is the principle that practitioners who function as experts must have the requisite experience in and knowledge about the clinical practice area. I caution you against "overreaching". Your credibility, if not your integrity, ultimately will be damaged if you venture outside the confines of your true expertise.

Second, never compromise your opinions for the sake of a case. Always remain true to the standard of care that you recognize as applicable to a given set of circumstances. As you know, a standard of care may require strict compliance with a narrowly defined treatment regimen in certain instances and may allow broad discretion in recommending alternative treatments in other instances. In the first instance, compliance with or deviation from the standard of care may be more obvious than in the second. In either situation, however, do not loosen the applicable standard to accommodate a litigant. Identify the relevant standard and apply it uniformly to each similar case. Serve only as an impartial third-party examiner, never as an advocate or partisan.

Of course, there may be situations where the standard of care by which you guide your own behavior is more strict than that followed by practitioners generally. Recognize this fact when you are called upon to assess a defendant's actions and employ the standard that applies to the profession as a whole. In this regard, keep in mind that many of the organizational pronouncements referred to earlier properly distinguish between malpractice and maloccurrence, that is, a bad result from proper treatment. Of course, this difference must be appreciated by anyone who offers to serve as a malpractice expert.

As mentioned previously, most experienced malpractice attorneys maintain and update databases about malpractice experts. Defense expert reports and testimony (deposition and trial) are stored and exchanged by members of the plaintiff's bar and are available for review and comparison. Defense attorneys engage in the same exercise. Consequently, if you have offered an opinion in a case that is decidedly different from that expressed on the same issue in another matter, the likelihood is that the adverse attorney will find it and attempt to use it to impeach your credibility. If the inconsistency results from truly different fact patterns, an "institutional" reassessment of the issue by the profession, or changed views prompted by new research, such inconsistencies will be easily explained. If not, your inconsistent opinions will be your undoing.

I represented an obstetrician whose alleged malpractice occurred in connection with the vaginal delivery of a baby during which shoulder dystocia was encountered. That is, one of the shoulders impacted against the mother's pubic bone preventing delivery. My client initially utilized gentle downward traction on the fetal head as well as other recognized maneuvers to dislodge the infant. Ultimately, the baby was delivered, but with a brachial plexus injury and an eventual diagnosis of Erb's Palsy with associated neurologic deficits in one of the infant's upper extremities. The plaintiff's obstetrical expert maintained that the improper application of pressure on the fetal head was responsible for the child's condition.

Prior to trial, I obtained copies of reports authored by the plaintiff's expert in matters where he had served as a defense expert. In one of those reports, the expert had defended the very conduct that he was now criticizing. At trial, I effectively confronted him with his inconsistent positions and irreparably damaged his credibility. When the jury returned its verdict, my client prevailed.

As noted, you should be familiar with the professional statements regarding expert service and the guidelines of behavior that they recite. Specific qualifications, like board certification, have been recommended as prerequisites by organizations if one intends to function as a malpractice expert. Stressed too is the need for truthful testimony about the standard of care. Typically, practitioners are also reminded that opinions offered in the context of a public proceeding, such as a malpractice lawsuit, are subject to scrutiny by the expert's peers. These guidelines emphasize that less than honest testimony may prompt a disciplinary, civil and/or criminal investigation.

In fact, state licensing boards are known to vigorously investigate complaints filed against practitioners who violate state statutory codes of conduct when serving as malpractice experts. For example, the New Jersey State Board of Medical Examiners can discipline a physician under *N.J.S.A.* 45:1–21e for "professional or occupational misconduct" and has done so where a medical malpractice expert's testimony concerning the standard of care was offered without sufficient knowledge.

The American Medical Association has issued a medical ethics opinion supporting its members' participation in the legal process and recognizing the expert's legitimate role in the promotion of justice. Others expressly acknowledge that experts should be paid for their services but advise that fees must be reasonable. Uniformly and unequivocally, they warn that fees should never be contingent; that is, they must never be based on the outcome of the litigation. Any such arrangement has been identified as unethical by the organizations that have addressed the issue.

Organizations such as the American Academy of Orthopaedic Surgeons and the American Society of General Surgeons have initiated expert witness programs that establish strict guidelines for expert service. Both have created an oath or affirmation to be signed by its members who serve as expert witnesses declaring adherence to principles of professionalism as have the American College of Surgeons and the American Urological Association. The American Society of General Surgeons has even adopted a Certification Program which encourages its members to become certified as expert witnesses upon satisfaction of certain identified requirements, including completion of an approved expert witness course, letters of recommendation and continuing medical education.

Never forget that the energy with which you approach expert service generally and with which you tackle each case specifically must be tempered by unwavering adherence to the applicable rules of behavior, however defined and interpreted by your profession and enforced by your state's licensing agency. Strict compliance should always be your guide. Be careful to avoid the ethical and legal pitfalls of getting involved in cases that prompt you to "push the envelope" too far. You will never be hurt professionally or personally if you refuse to compromise your integrity. In fact, your "cachet" will only be enhanced as your reputation develops as a reliable, consistent and straight-shooting expert.

Chapter 11

Accepting the Challenge

Little more needs to be said about how to succeed as a defense expert in malpractice matters. Your expert career can provide you with satisfaction on many levels. As with anything worthwhile, development as an expert requires time, effort and attention. However, once you capably handle that first assignment, others will follow, and with each new matter, your experience will grow and your reputation will blossom.

Remember. An experienced and modestly busy expert may receive between 15 and 20 files a years or more, depending upon that expert's specialty. Each liability case accepted will force you to focus on standard of care issues. It also will give you the opportunity to impact the malpractice environment generally by participating in malpractice matters in a mean-ingful way. No matter the jurisdiction and the protections afforded malpractice defendants under its laws, our country's legal system affords patients the right to file suit for alleged malpractice. As a result, there will always be a need for mal-practice defense experts. Since I am certain the "better" the expert, the better the chance for trial success, quality practitio-ners determined to address a hostile malpractice environment can affect the system in a powerful fashion from within, by serving as defense experts.

The point is the defense of malpractice claims will only benefit from an increase in the number of available and competent expert witnesses. Certainly, defense attorneys will welcome the help of more well-credentialed practitioners who have a real interest in expert work and who have or can develop a facility to capably function in the litigation arena. There can be little downside to exploring the possibilities, and since you now know what it takes to succeed as a malpractice defense expert, why not accept the challenge?

Printed in the United States
by Baker & Taylor Publisher Services